The Plan Cookbook

the **Plan**

COOKBOOK

More Than 150 Recipes for
Vibrant Health and Weight Loss

Lyn-Genet Recitas

New York Times
bestselling author of
The Plan

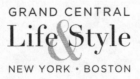

GRAND CENTRAL
Life & Style
NEW YORK · BOSTON

Grand Central Life & Style
Hachette Book Group
1290 Avenue of the Americas
New York, NY 10104

www.GrandCentralLifeandStyle.com

Printed in the United States of America

RRD-C

First Edition: December 2014
10 9 8 7 6 5 4 3 2 1

Grand Central Life & Style is an imprint of Grand Central Publishing.
The Grand Central Life & Style name and logo are trademarks of Hachette Book Group, Inc.

The Hachette Speakers Bureau provides a wide range of authors for speaking events. To find out more, go to www.HachetteSpeakersBureau.com or call (866) 376-6591.

The publisher is not responsible for websites (or their content) that are not owned by the publisher.

Library of Congress Cataloging-in-Publication Data

Recitas, Lyn-Genet.
  The plan cookbook : More than 150 delicious recipes for vibrant health and weight loss / Lyn-Genet Recitas, *New York Times* bestselling author of the plan. — First edition.
     pages cm
  Includes bibliographical references and index.
  ISBN 978-1-4555-5653-3 (hardback) — ISBN 978-1-4555-5652-6 (ebook)   1. Weight loss—Health aspects.
2. Body weight—Health aspects.   3. Nutrition.   4. Reducing diets—Recipes.   5. Self-care, Health.   I. Title.
  RM222.2.R425 2015
  613.2'5—dc23
                                                                                                                              2014017847

First and foremost this book is dedicated to my family: Thank you always, Bill, for your love and patience; to my son, Brayden, who lights up my heart and cracks me up; to Ella, who has taught me how much food can heal; and to Ted Recitas, for always being such a great, true friend.

Contents

The Plan
Cookbook

CHAPTER 1

Inflammation

The Hidden Cause of Weight Gain

Samantha, 43

I finished twenty days of The Plan and lost twelve pounds! The Plan is amazing! It is like it was written just for me....I had thyroid cancer, Lyme disease, acid reflux, night sweats, and a host of medical issues. Before The Plan I ate healthy and exercised, yet was always sick, tired, and couldn't lose weight no matter what I did. But not with The Plan—I love it! Thank you so much! The book changed my life and I'm sharing it with everyone!

Jack, 35

I just completed the first twenty days of The Plan this weekend. I just want to say thank you, Lyn-Genet. You have changed my life! I am thirty-five years old and for the last year I have suffered from severe allergies. The doctors had me on steroids that caused me to put on extra weight. I also suffer from knee joint pain and the extra weight was causing serious flare-ups. I always felt I was too young to feel like this, but I didn't know what to do about it. After twenty days on The Plan, I can honestly say I feel the best I have felt in the last year. I feel like me again. The joint pain, gone. Allergies under control. I lost eighteen pounds and I'm learning to love new foods like kale and lamb that I can stick to the rest of my life. You are truly a lifesaver! Thank you!

These testimonials are just a sampling of the hundreds of thousands I've heard since my book *The Plan* landed on the shelves in January 2013. Suddenly, people like Samantha and Jack have been able to take weight off that's been stuck to them for years and change their health. In just twenty days. People feel healthier, more energetic, and more clearheaded than they have in years. All because they've learned what foods work, and don't work, for them.

Now, I know what you're thinking. "I know what to eat already. I only eat the healthiest foods. It's just that sometimes I get lazy and have some fun foods or don't get to the gym enough. That's why I'm putting on weight. My metabolism just isn't what it used to be."

What if I told you it probably isn't the fun foods and you don't have to work out as much as you think to be in the best shape and weight in your life? The truth of the matter is that what you think you should be eating may well be the wrong foods. And the foods you think you should be avoiding? They may not be the problem at all.

It's not about eating the foods you've been told are healthy. Instead, it's about finding the foods that work for your unique chemistry. To simplify, what's healthy for me may not be healthy for you. How many times have you stepped on a scale after a "healthy" day and wondered how you *gained* weight? Or eaten healthy foods but wound up feeling bloated and constipated? Why are you trying so hard and gaining weight and feeling sicker?

The answer is simple: No food is healthy if it causes inflammation for you. If you are eating foods that don't work for your body's chemistry, you won't lose weight—in fact, you'll wind up feeling worse and gaining weight.

The Easy Way to Lose Weight

Traditional diets—the diets that you're used to, like no carb, unlimited protein, low fat, or calorie counting—don't work because there is no universal one-size-fits-all solution when it comes to weight loss. These diets are promoting what they think are healthy foods, but that's a major problem because there's no such thing as universally "healthy" foods, especially for those over the age of thirty-five.

When you eat a food that doesn't work for your body, it triggers an inflammatory response. This response affects your waistline and your immune system, and hastens the aging process. The Plan works by taking those foods out of the equation. When you're no longer eating those foods, you lower chronic low-grade inflammation and everything falls into place. Your weight, your health, and your mood all balance, like you always knew they could.

Ironically, some of the most reactive foods are considered to be some of the top diet foods. They include:

- Asparagus
- Black beans
- Cauliflower
- Greek yogurt
- Oatmeal
- Salmon
- Turkey

I know you're probably having a tough time believing that foods like oatmeal and salmon can make anyone fat. But here's the reality. Each person is chemically unique. Certain foods may work for a large population, but when combined with your individual chemistry, they can be toxic. This does *not* mean the foods I just listed are bad for you—there is no good, there is no bad. Instead, certain foods work with your body's chemistry and others don't. The beauty of the recipes that you'll find in this book is that they work well for the chemistry of most people. We've had hundreds of thousands of people test these foods, all while lowering inflammation and normalizing thyroid function.

Shonda, 51, and Jerome, 56

The Plan was a lifesaver! I was at risk for type 2 diabetes and my cholesterol was 246 and triglycerides were 194. Since starting The Plan, I have lost sixty-six pounds and my husband has lost eighty-three pounds. My cholesterol is down to 163 and my triglycerides are 112. I feel good enough to exercise and my joint pain has gone away. We love the food so much, this doesn't even feel like a diet. I know this has saved me from a lifetime of taking medications!

Eating to Tame the Flame

Inflammation is big news today. You see it on television shows and read about it in newspapers, magazines, and medical journals. And there's a good reason it's so ever present in the news. Inflammation is a big problem; it makes you sick and old, and causes weight gain.

I'll explain in more detail about the dangers of inflammation later, but for now, let's just say that inflammation—a physiological process that can help you heal—can also lead to a host of problems. Chronic inflammation exacerbates and hastens the aging process because it floods tissue with free radicals and promotes the destruction of normal cells. Research shows that chronic inflammation is also a major contributor to the aging of the cardiovascular and nervous systems. Inflammation is now recognized as one of the key risk factors for heart disease, diabetes, high cholesterol, stroke, and cognitive and neurological disorders.

The immune system's response to an inflammatory diet diverts the body's energy from healing and repair and allows whatever is latent in our genetic makeup to kick up whatever is chronic and worsen it. (See "Are You Suffering from Food-Induced Inflammation?" on page 6 for a list of a few of those conditions.)

There's one other very notable result of inflammation: weight gain. Until The Plan came out, no one had said that foods cause inflammation, but I've seen and charted this effect for years with my clients. Eat a food that doesn't work for your body and the next day you are up a pound or more. I have seen a four-pound weight gain in one day from one inflammatory food! These foods cause such an instant reaction in your body that I call them *reactive foods*.

Janet, 48

I had been diagnosed with lupus, Crohn's, depression, and hypothyroidism. Then in March 2013, I got *The Plan* and started focusing on what I was putting in my body, keeping a daily food journal and tracking my food responses. I have lost a total of fifty-one pounds in ten months, going from 177 pounds to 126 pounds. I no longer take pain or anxiety medication and am down to taking just one pill a day. Thank you!

Listen to Your Body

When I opened up my health center eight years ago in New York, I communicated with my clients on a weekly basis. Like most nutritionists, I'd tell my clients to eat healthy foods, and when they gained weight or didn't lose fast enough, we both thought it was because of the "fun foods" they'd indulged in during the week. The cheeseburger and fries that you had as a treat were obviously a big problem when it came to losing weight, right? It turns out that that wasn't the problem, and like everyone else, I had a few ideas that were totally wrong.

Once the BlackBerry came along, I urged my clients to pop me regular daily emails, and those weekly appointments turned into hourly updates. I'd get an email from a client *immediately* after they ate a food that wasn't right for them. Bam! Their bodies would react like lit gunpowder, firing up in an instant. That's when I started to realize that weight was much more than a calories-in, calories-out equation. Two clients could eat the same food and have completely different responses. If a client ate something that didn't agree with their chemistry, they would experience gas, bloating, stuffy nose, joint pain, migraines, depression, and/or digestive issues—within minutes of eating the reactive food. These minute-by-minute updates allowed me to track information and start to see a definite pattern. The wrong food will kick-start health issues, and the next day that number on the scale will jump up.

I quickly came to realize that what I had always believed was healthy wasn't holding water when it came to clients, so I started to track individual responses to so-called "healthy" foods. I noticed that 85 percent of my clients reacted to black beans, 85 percent reacted to salmon. This was mind-boggling to me. What was really fascinating was that these responses were more than just weight gain—clients were showing clear signs of inflammation, whether in the form of fatigue, digestive issues, joint pain, or other ill effects. I had been studying inflammation and its effects on the body and kept scouring the research to see what I could find on whether specific foods can cause weight gain and inflammation. Despite the fact that I couldn't find this in the published research, I was seeing it daily with my eyes. Eat a food that doesn't work for you, and you gain weight and get sick. I was blown away as I realized that so many foods I believed were health promoting were the exact opposite.

Are You Suffering from Food-Induced Inflammation?

These are common reactions to inflammatory foods:

- Allergies
- Arthritis
- Bloating
- Constipation
- Depression

- Diarrhea
- Exhaustion
- Headaches
- Hormonal imbalance

- Irritability
- Joint pain
- Sinusitis
- Skin conditions
- Sleeplessness

These reactions are actually your body's way of saying, "Please don't feed this food to me!" Your body is recognizing this food as the "bad guy" and the immune system launches an instantaneous attack. While this attack is happening, the body's instinct to repair takes a back seat and can only restart when this danger is resolved. This is how we can get sick. You see, the body always wants to operate in perfect balance, repairing and healing. This is called *homeostasis*. But when there's a fire, the body is going to deal with the flames first, and ignore the rest of the body's systems.

The immune system's response to an inflammatory diet diverts the body's energy from healing and repair and allows whatever is latent in our genetic makeup to spring forth, like high cholesterol, diabetes, and heart disease. But you can stop this cycle. Just by changing what you eat.

Calories—Stop Counting Them

I'm going to tell you something that you've probably never heard. But this concept has helped hundreds of thousands lose weight more quickly and easily than they ever thought possible.

You've no doubt been told that the only way you can lose weight is to cut calories. But that simply isn't true. Because losing weight is not about how many calories you're taking in. In fact, losing weight has nothing to do with calories at all. That's right, losing weight has nothing do with calories.

Weight gain can be attributed to a few basic issues:

- You're not drinking enough water.
- You're eating too much sodium.
- You eat foods that are reactive.
- You exercise too much.
- You are too stressed out.

You've probably noticed that eating too many calories isn't on that list! Nice!

This book will give you helpful tools and tips to manage these factors and, of course, dozens of low-reactive, low-sodium recipes that will help you lose weight and feel terrific. All without counting a single calorie.

Yes, you can get the healthy body you've always dreamed of, and you don't have to starve yourself to do it. In fact, when you eliminate foods that are reactive you can actually eat *more,* because your body is no longer experiencing the responses that hinder digestion. Hinder digestion, gain weight. It's that simple.

Inflammation and Weight Gain

Many people think the reason we gain weight as we get older is because our metabolism is slowing down. And there is some truth to that. But the main factor for weight gain as we age is that our body loses digestive enzymes and stomach acid, and even saliva decreases! So some of the foods we were able to eat in our twenties become problematic in our thirties, forties, and fifties. This is also the time when we start to have health issues, especially digestive issues.

Here's a story I use to explain how a healthy food can wreak havoc with our waistlines. I like to use green beans in this story because they're a food that's universally thought of as healthy.

Let's say you eat 100 calories of green beans when you're twenty. At that age, odds are you're at your digestive peak and those green-bean calories will most likely burn off just the same as they did coming in. Calories in = calories out. By the time you reach twenty-five, those 100 calories of green beans will start acting like 200 calories. But you can moderate weight gain by eating a little healthier, working out a little more, and beginning the latest diet craze.

Then you get to age thirty-five...a major inflammatory speed bump. And suddenly, that 100 calories of green beans start to act like 700 calories. By the time you're forty-two, they act like 3,500 calories; by the time you reach fifty, they act like 7,000 calories! But wait a minute. How can 100 calories of green beans act like 7,000 calories? That's where inflammation comes in.

Look to Your Gut

Did you know that 60 to 70 percent of your immune system is in your gut? GALT, or gut associated lymphoid tissue, contains 70 percent of your immune system and is located in your gastrointestinal tract. It moderates responses to bacteria, viruses, and pathogens and has receptors ready to attack within minutes of contact with anything foreign—and with "normal" substances that are deemed as foreign! This triggers the release of our body's defense crew, like natural killer cells, cytokines, and interferon, to name a few.

I'm going to explain this to you in more detail in the next chapter, but for now, here's what you need to know. Food sensitivity is an example of how weight and health are triggered by a reactive food. Perhaps you're familiar with the term *histamine*? You've probably heard it in the context of seasonal allergies. Histamine is an important part of our immune system because it springs into action when a person is exposed to something he's allergic or sensitive to.

The immune system is designed to protect your body against foreign substances. In the case of allergies, the body thinks that an airborne substance (like pollen or dander) is harmful. The immune system of the allergic person, thinking that this allergen is going to cause harm, tries to mobilize and attack by releasing histamine and other chemicals into the body. The histamine then acts on a person's eyes, nose, throat, lungs, skin, or gastrointestinal tract, causing those notoriously unpleasant allergy symptoms.

Histamine is also triggered when an inflammatory food is introduced. Histamine causes water retention by causing capillaries to dilate and allowing them to leak fluid, so you'll see an immediate gain on the scale when you eat an inflammatory food. But the inflammatory response is not *just* water weight. Water weight can be reversed within twenty-four hours. A reactive response can easily last for seventy-two hours and it causes more than just weight gain. Eating a food that doesn't work for your body can kick-start *any* latent health issues you have (think constipation, acid reflux, IBS, and so on).

To control this histamine response, the body produces cortisol. Cortisol and hormones such as progesterone and testosterone use the same building blocks; the more cortisol that is released, the more your hormonal balance is negatively affected. The body is producing cortisol at the expense of progesterone and testosterone. These hormonal fluctuations disrupt water balance, metabolism, thyroid health, healthy sex drive, and immune response. Elevated cortisol raises glucose, which leads to increased blood sugar levels. This will start to increase yeast growth as it has specialized glucose sensors, and its growth in population will alter gut flora affecting your body's defense system. A high yeast population means never-ending sugar and carb cravings (and high sugar and carb intake is definitely a factor behind the incredible rise of type 2 diabetes in the US). Altered gut flora leads to a weakened immune response as the balance of our intestinal bacteria is thrown off.

This might sound amazing to you, but yes: Every time you eat a food that doesn't work for you this whole system gets started. There are other factors of course. Certain foods known as *goitrogens* attack thyroid function (I'll explain more about that in Chapter 2), but the diagram below gives you a basic idea of what happens when you eat a food that is reactive.

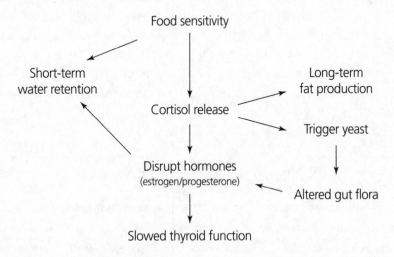

Here's what happens in your body when you eat a reactive food.

Sarai, 44

When I compliment my friends on how great they look after they lose weight, I hear from far too many of them that they "don't eat much." I used to be one of them, until that kind of dieting stopped working for me in my forties. I gained fifteen to twenty pounds and was following a restrictive 1,200-to-1,400-calorie-a-day diet. I worked out five or six times a week for one to one and a half hours and was practically vegan with a bit of fish (only wild and locally caught). I watched my friends on the same diet dropping weight, but my acne, PMS, and hypothyroidism continued and I only lost eight pounds, which I worked hard to maintain with my low-calorie diet and workout schedule. I was exhausted! And beyond frustrated.

And then The Plan entered my life. All of a sudden, I was able to eat so much food, and all different types of food—so much food that I could not seem to finish a meal on The Plan!

I was skeptical because I had tried it all: Weight Watchers, Medifast, vegan, vegetarian, pescatarian, all organic, lots of exercise, no exercise—all of them started great and ended with weight gain. Taking one more chance, I committed to The Plan with the same loyal, honest commitment I had given to the others. And I lost weight. . . . *Fast!* Five pounds the first week, and it just kept coming. I was losing weight daily. I ate foods I had cut out (with trepidation, but I did it), I had wine and chocolate every night, ate gourmet meals that were fast to prepare, cheese, potato chips, bread—foods I'd avoided for years! And yet I dropped ten pounds in twenty days! It turns out wild white fish, scallops, sun-dried tomatoes, and hummus (which I ate daily for protein) were causing me to gain weight. I cut those out and have kept the weight off, without *ever* counting calories. Not only that, but I am medication free when I eat Plan menus consistently. Amazing! Miraculous! It is only twenty days; you can do anything for twenty days. Commit and do your best to do it 100 percent and it will happen for you!

I'll Never Lose Weight; It's My Genes

If you don't remember a time when you weren't chubby, you may have just been born with weaker digestion. In fact, we see many people who had seasonal, food, and environmental allergies as a child and now, as adults, have a tendency to be overweight. It can take several generations to build up enzymes for the genetic mutations in our food, so if you or your parents are new to the States there's a good chance you aren't digesting your food as well as your peers. Remember, poor digestion usually means weight gain, allergies, and health issues. Having constantly heightened levels of histamine means your body is always ready to explode in response to a reactive food.

The first thing I ask clients who tell me they've always been overweight is, "Did you have strong seasonal, environmental allergies or asthma as a child?" Not surprisingly, the answer is often yes. I cannot tell you what a sigh of relief everyone lets out when I tell them their wiring is more sensitive than most people's. These poor people have been beating themselves up their whole lives just because their wiring is off! But it's not their fault! You wouldn't beat yourself up for having curly or straight hair, would you? Well, it's the same for digestive strength. That was the way your body used to work and we are going to change that.

The good news is we can lower histamine levels and strengthen your gut. It just takes the right foods and a bit of short-term help with supplements like MSM (see page 17) and probiotics, which we will discuss at length later. These supplements will prime your body to digest food better and to lessen internal stress on your body.

Your Thyroid—A Fountain of Vitality

The thyroid, which we will discuss in the next chapter, is responsible for every metabolic and cellular activity. What's amazing is that the thyroid only produces 1 teaspoon of thyroid hormone a year! So you can quickly understand that anything that interferes with its functioning can affect you on every level.

So much of thyroid dysfunction is based on reactive foods, heightened levels of cortisol, and nutritional deficiencies. If we can control these factors, we can restore thyroid functioning and help our bodies operate at 110 percent. Think of the thyroid as the key unlocking each function in your body! Eat the right foods, boost your thyroid function, and you'll feel and look the best you ever have.

Oh, and another bonus? With the right foods, you'll be boosting your sex drive. You have no idea how many women say to me, "I love my husband but I never want to touch the guy! I have no sex drive and by the end of the day I am so exhausted!" Well, it takes a lot of energy to digest reactive foods. It also doesn't help that many of the foods attack thyroid function. So packing on the pounds and having low energy and no sex drive all too often becomes the norm for many of us in our forties and on. Women and men are beating themselves up when they can switch the cycle by eating foods that work for their chemistry.

Benita, 51

Between three kids, working full-time, and all the extra weight I had been carrying, the last thing I wanted to do was go on a date with my husband. I felt tired, unsexy, and had a really short fuse. After following The Plan, I felt good again—I was down eighteen and a half pounds, had more energy, and wasn't as easily irritated! Recently my husband and I went out to a new restaurant together—it was the most fun we have had in literally years. I couldn't believe how much I was laughing, and my husband kept saying how great I looked. It was so nice to feel romantic and make out like teenagers. I feel like a new woman and am so glad I did this!

How This Book Can Help

There are two crucial steps to achieving the healthy, feel-good, look-great body you have always wanted.

1. RESET YOUR SYSTEM

Eating foods that work well with your body enables it to reach homeostasis, a state of stability and repair. In this book you will learn the steps of a three-day cleanse in which you eat the foods I have found to be non- or low reactive, such as blueberries, chicken, rice, and broccoli. If you've already done The Plan, you know which foods work best for you. If you haven't done The Plan, I highly recommend going through the twenty days and finding the foods that make you 110 percent *you*. However, that's not a requirement. All the recipes in this book contain the foods I've found to be the least inflammatory and are chock-full of ingredients that promote thyroid health.

2. WE'RE GOING TO CUSTOMIZE YOUR CUISINE

You will learn how to quickly put together delicious easy-to-prepare meals that fill you up and fuel your day. The whole family gets on The Plan, so making separate dinners

Nutrients That Support the Thyroid

If you follow the recipes in this book, you will be getting the nutrients you need to keep your thyroid healthy. I don't recommend taking any supplement for an extended period of time. Why take pills and waste money when you can get everything you need from food?

Zinc, found in lamb, pumpkin seeds
Vitamin B12, found in animal protein
Iodine, found in halibut, flounder, scallops, crab (low-reactive fish and seafood)
Vitamin A, found in kale, carrots, cayenne, chili peppers, butternut squash
Selenium, found in lamb, halibut, flounder, sunflower seeds
Vitamin E, found in sunflower seeds, almonds, kale, broccoli
Iron, found in kale, animal protein, beets

for you, the kids, and your spouse is not how we roll. Trust me, your family won't complain when you serve them the delicious recipes in this book! I know you're busy, so whether you are single and cooking for one or a busy parent working two jobs, this food will nourish you without straining your budget or sucking up all of your time.

Amanda, 43

I went to see a naturopathic doctor because I thought I was suffering from undiagnosed thyroid issues and I couldn't get my general practitioner to listen to my concerns. My naturopathic doctor recommended The Plan. I was so exhausted, I really didn't think I had the energy to try the diet, but I didn't know how much longer I could carry on being the tired mom of four young children. My husband started The Plan with me in solidarity, and within the first three days of the cleanse I started to notice a difference. Swelling was down in my face and I felt more alive, more awake, and more energized. So far I have lost about seventeen pounds and he has lost fifteen. Last week on the way to a wedding I realized, I'm happy. Happy. I'd always known in my mind I should be happy with four great kids and a loving husband, but I never felt it. Now I do. No, not just happy...I feel *great*! Thank you for this program. I think it is saving my life.

The Plan turns everything you have learned about food and health upside down. All that matters for your health and a healthy weight is eating the foods that work for your unique chemistry. Your low-inflammatory foods, your friendly foods, are the foods that work to support your health. These are the foods that will have you dancing on a table at your grandchild's wedding.

In the next few chapters, I'll walk you through some additional information that will be helpful as you start to follow (or continue to follow) this powerful program. I'll go into supplements, outline the basics of my three-day cleanse that will jump-start your journey to health, and discuss some of the most common diet trends that are out there.

In chapters 6 through 11 of this book, you'll find all of the recipes you need to live The Plan for life and enjoy every delicious moment of it. This program is not about deprivation. Not only will you be eating plenty of food—over 2,000 calories a day for women and over 2,800 calories a day for men—but you'll be eating delicious food: the kinds of meals that will please the whole family. Whether you eat paleo, vegetarian, gluten free, or just like a good burger or burrito, this book provides the healthiest, least inflammatory recipes. If you've spent years trying to diet and follow restrictive programs only to find that you're getting heavier and feeling sicker, this book will open your eyes to a new way of living and enjoying food. You'll lose weight and gain energy while enjoying delicious meals like Healthy Chicken Parmesan (page 167), Butternut Squash–Chicken "Tostadas" (page 170), and Chicken Pad Thai with Zucchini Pasta (page 166). *Bon appétit!*

CHAPTER 2

The Plan

Hormones, Hunger, and Health

The Plan isn't a diet. It's a complete change of mind-set. What you learn in this book may radically change the way you look at food, and the recipes will put that knowledge into practice and onto your plate!

In my practice, I've met so many people who were eating well yet still packing on the pounds, all because they were eating reactive foods that caused inflammation. Each person's response to healthy foods is different. This is known as bio-individuality. For instance, I'm super reactive to eggs. I eat *one* 70-calorie egg and I look six months pregnant, I'll gain a pound, and my sinuses will flare up. In the meantime, you may be able to eat scrambled eggs a few times a week, lose weight, and feel great.

Some of this is dictated by genetics. For instance, if you have Northern European roots, your body has developed the digestive enzymes to break down cow's milk cheese, which was a major food source in that region for millennia. If you have Asian or African roots? Not so much. Overconsumption of a food can produce allergies and so sesame seed allergies are higher in Israel and other parts of the Middle East. Rice allergies? Pretty high in China and Japan. So, there are genetic and cultural eating differences that make this puzzle much more interesting, too!

I have had emails and letters from people all over the world thanking me for confirming their suspicions: Certain foods made them feel unwell. The Plan teaches you to start trusting your gut again and stop letting health experts dictate which foods you eat. As one man told me, "It's not rocket science. Every time I ate pork I gained a pound and felt like garbage. So I stopped eating pork!"

In The Plan, I walk you through a detailed program that starts with a three-day cleanse designed to heal and reset the body. The foods you eat during those three days are universally tolerated, so right away we bring down the level of inflammation in your body and set you on track to lose weight and start feeling better. From there, you will introduce different foods, one at a time, to see how that food reacts in your body.

Most people have a very strong reaction to a food that's reactive—they feel sleepy, or bloated or gassy, and the next day the number on the scale ticks up. The whole program is your scientific experiment to determine the ideal diet for your body. And, as you've heard through some of the testimonials sprinkled throughout this book, the results have been extraordinary!

Alan, 55

I have had multiple sclerosis since 2001. Since MS is an autoimmune disease, the less active your immune system is, the better. I picked up a copy of *The Plan* thinking that if I can find the foods that will not cause my immune system to act up, I might feel better. So far, I have lost more than twenty-five pounds. I feel great and my MS symptoms have been pretty quiet. I'm an ex-Olympic athlete and was in the Los Angeles Olympics in 1984. For the first time in a long time, I can now ride a bike for fifty miles!

Where Should I Start?

In this book, I share over 150 recipes that contain the foods I've found to be the least inflammatory overall. These are the foods that most people can tolerate well and that don't cause a bad reaction. But, as you now know, you may react differently to a food! Some of these low-inflammatory foods might not be optimal for you and that's not what we want!

So here's my best advice for readers that are new to this philosophy and want to dive right in. Start with the three-day cleanse that begins on page 45. Then try the recipes in the book and just note how you feel. Does your energy dip after a meal, are you gassy and bloated, do your sinuses clog? Try to avoid those foods. Do meals make you feel fantastic, is your stomach flat, your mood and digestion great? Put those foods in your friendly food arsenal!

For a bit more guidance, the chart on page 18 shows the reactivity potential of many of the most common foods. This chart is based on years of experience and hands-on research with thousands of clients. The rates are based on the percentage of our clients who test reactive to these foods.

Supplements and Medications

I get a lot of questions from readers and clients about supplements and medication. Many people want to know if they should stop taking their supplements and medications when they begin The Plan.

All in all, I am not a big believer in supplements, and I only recommend them as a short-term catalyst to get the body's functions going. After everything's humming along smoothly, I recommend you discontinue regular use and take them only on an as-needed basis.

For example, when I start feeling a sniffle coming on, I'll take zinc. As soon as I feel better, the zinc goes back in the fridge. A big joke in our office is that on Mondays, the staff and I take SAM-e (see page 19) to deal with Monday morning stress. Then on Tuesday morning, the bottle goes back in the cabinet.

Our most recommended supplements are MSM, SAM-e, probiotics, a good liver cleanser like milk thistle for your first twenty days on The Plan, and a thyroid supplement like kelp and B12 if your BBT (basal body temperature) is consistently below 96. MSM is usually taken for six weeks to reduce histamine and boost mucosal strength. Probiotics should only be taken on an as-needed basis, such as if you have gas, bloating, or constipation and when yeast kicks up (the biggest telltale sign is a white-coated tongue).

MSM: Strengthening Your Mucosa

MSM (methylsulfonylmethane) is a histamine inhibitor that helps to alleviate food, environmental, and seasonal allergies by strengthening mucosae (mucous membranes). My team and I at The Plan find it especially helpful for healing sinus, esophageal, lung, and intestinal mucosa.

REACTIVE FOODS

Highly Reactive

85%+ Reactive
Shrimp
Farm-raised fish
Turkey
Tomato sauce
Eggplant
Oatmeal
Greek yogurt
Black beans
Cannellini beans
Cauliflower
Cabbage
Hard-boiled eggs
Non-organic spinach
Salmon

Asparagus
Corn
Bagels
Roasted nut butter and nuts
Deli meats
Veal
Sushi

70% Reactive
Regular yogurt
Green beans
Pork
Pasta
Bananas
Canned tomatoes

Tomato sauce

60% Reactive
Peppers
Mushrooms (excluding shiitake, maitake, and enoki)
Cod
Tuna
Pineapple
Grapefruit
Artichokes
Quinoa
Strawberries
Oranges
Almond milk

Medium Reactive

50% Reactive
Cow's milk
Couscous
White rice
Tomatoes
Edamame
Peas
Tahini

40% Reactive
Wild white fish
Lentils

Pintos
Peas
Lactose-free milk
Whole eggs

30% Reactive
Wild flounder, halibut
Egg whites
Bok choy
Cow's milk cheese
Sunflower butter
Crab (except Alaskan king crab)

Lobster

20% Reactive
Wheat
Scallops
Brussels sprouts
Snow peas
Winter squash
Salmon sashimi and yellowtail
Sesame seeds
Tempeh
Kamut, spelt

Low Reactive

10% Reactive
Potatoes (in small amounts)
Duck
Hemp seeds

5% or Less Reactive
Avocados
Mangos
Beef
Garlic
Chickpeas
Onions

Shiitake mushrooms (may be higher if you have systemic yeast)
Radicchio
Endive
Lamb
Chicken
Goat or sheep's cheese
Pears
Broccoli
Carrots
Kale

Zucchini
Beets
Sunflower seeds
Pumpkin seeds
Raw almonds
Apples
Blueberries
Rice cereal
Chia seeds
Frisee
Coconut milk
Rice milk

MSM can be used to alleviate:

- Allergies
- Acid reflux
- Asthma
- Arthritis
- Inflammation (especially of mucous membranes)
- Migraines

It can also help to boost collagen production, assist in liver detoxification, and restore gut function.

Therapeutic doses of MSM range from 3,000 to 6,000 milligrams. A dose of 3,000 milligrams works best for people up to 180 pounds; 4,000 milligrams for people up to 240 pounds; 5,000 milligrams for people up to 320 pounds; and 6,000 milligrams for people who are over 400 pounds. Always check with your doctor before taking any supplements.

SAM-e: Your Stress Buddy

SAM-e is a supplement that is amazing during times of stress. Heightened levels of cortisol (the hormone released during periods of stress) will affect your hormones, thyroid, and weight. I may not be able to change the stress in your life, but SAM-e can certainly mitigate your response to it!

SAM-e stands for S-adenosyl methionine and is made in the body from a reaction between methionine, an amino acid, and ATP, which is an energy molecule. SAM-e is involved in many different reactions in the body and levels drop as we age. It has been used to treat depression, liver problems, fibromyalgia, musculoskeletal pain, and arthritis. Many women use it for hormonal problems including PMS and perimenopause. It has been shown to increase levels of serotonin, also known as the feel-good hormone because it plays an essential role in warding off depression and boosting mood. SAM-e is contraindicated for bipolar disorder and may interfere with Parkinson's medications, so check with your doctor before supplementing.

Always check with your doctor before taking SAM-e if you are on antidepressants and make sure you're under the care of a doctor if you decrease the dosage of your medications.

Arthur, 58

I was on Wellbutrin (an antidepressant) and had tried weaning off of it once before. I started following The Plan for a couple of months and after cutting out reactive foods and eating more healing foods, I felt better equipped to try again. I spoke to my doctor and I started to taper off my meds. Using SAM-e for a few weeks really helped! Now I only take it on stressful days and during work deadlines. I'm now down thirty-eight pounds and have such a positive attitude. I was also able to completely eliminate my blood pressure meds. People around me can barely recognize that I'm the same person!

Probiotics: For a Healthy Gut

We also rotate in probiotics to restore your gastrointestinal balance when you eat a reactive food or when your yeast kicks up. As soon as you start to experience any bloating or gas, a probiotic will help to alleviate discomfort and weight gain.

Liver Cleanser

To optimize healing during your first twenty days on The Plan, I recommend a liver cleanser as the liver is responsible for over five hundred functions. Because we are exposed to so many environmental pollutants, pesticides, and chemicals, our livers can easily be overtaxed. The extra support from a liver supplement aids weight loss and hormonal balance, to name just a few really important functions. This can be as mild as dandelion tea or taken as a stronger supplement like milk thistle and dandelion extract.

Thyroid Help

A healthy thyroid is a key part of overall health and mood. Anything that disrupts thyroid function can have huge ramifications in every aspect of your life. A sluggish thyroid is often caused by nutritional deficiencies. Eating Plan friendly means better thyroid health as many of the nutrients needed to support its function are part of the diet. We will discuss later how you may want to introduce kelp and B12 supplements for a short time using your basal body temperature as your guide.

Should I Test for Food Allergies?

Another major question I get from readers and clients is whether or not they should test for food allergies or intolerances. The ALCAT test (antigen leukocyte antibody test) is one of the more popular tests that is used to diagnose food allergy or intolerance. Unfortunately, I find it very unreliable.

As I'll explain later in the book, if you don't rotate your foods and eat a varied diet, you'll build up sensitivity to them. If you eat a lot of a particular food right before your ALCAT test, it's going to show up as a bigger sensitivity. For example, if you eat chicken every day before your ALCAT test, you're going to show up as having a huge sensitivity to chicken when, in fact, you might be just fine with chicken in moderation. In addition, women will test more sensitive to foods if they have the ALCAT run when they're ovulating or five to seven days before their menstrual period. If you have seasonal allergies you may show as sensitive to more foods during allergy season. In fact there are so many variables that come into play with the ALCAT test that we at The Plan find it's not truly reflective of what's going on in your body.

Then we have the people who come to our clinic frustrated because all their favorite foods tested positive on the ALCAT, so they eat a totally new batch of foods without rotating them. Well, guess who is setting themselves up to build a new batch of food sensitivities?

At The Plan we like to say "Rotate or React." If you aren't rotating your foods, it's very easy to create a food sensitivity. When you keep eating the same foods there's a good chance that not all of the chemicals in the foods will agree with your body and they will start to overburden your body with problematic compounds. If you don't identify these food sensitivities, they can often turn into food allergies! Conversely, if you cut out a food that has been on the "no" list for a three-to-six-month period, there's a very good chance you will be able to eat it on occasion.

Maria, 39

I can't believe that so many of my favorite foods were reactive! But I took Lyn-Genet's advice to rotate foods and started retesting foods three months later. By the time I reached six months of eating Plan friendly, I felt like nothing was reactive anymore. I can even eat bread and cheese and lose weight! Best part is no more migraines. I would have done anything to stop them; I wish I would have done this years ago.

Get Ready to Lose

When I first wrote *The Plan,* people simply could not believe that a 100-calorie "healthy" food like green beans or a big bowl of piping hot oatmeal could cause a two-pound weight gain, and make them sick. But it can.

How? As I've explained in Chapter 1, the simplest answer is that certain foods set off an inflammatory response with your particular body chemistry. Many systems come into play with a reactive food and this causes the domino effect that we usually associate with getting older—think expanding waistline, lower energy, and declining health.

Let's start with some basics. Aging is, in and of itself, a state of inflammation. As we age, systems start to naturally slow down, including digestion. Production of digestive enzymes, stomach acid, and saliva—all key to proper food digestion—starts to slow down. The foods our bodies used to be able to break down easily become more difficult to digest. So these foods that used to fly through our systems when we were at our digestive peak now become trigger foods that affect our health and weight.

When you eat a food that your body is sensitive to, the immune system releases chemicals to attack what it thinks is an invader. Digestion is inhibited and this poor digestion impairs metabolism and endocrine function, causing your body to store fluids and fat. When you eat that food again and again, the body is continually forced to launch this immune response. It becomes overwhelmed and, in its weakened state, becomes even more sensitive to your reactive foods.

Once your body becomes overly reactive to a food, it's bad news for your weight no matter how many nutrients that food contains. I've mentioned green beans before, so let's use those as an example. If you're sensitive to green beans, your body thinks those green beans are the "bad guy," something foreign it needs to fight. Think about what happens when you're slicing up some tomatoes and you accidentally nick your finger. The injury triggers a cascade of events that brings more blood cells to the area. The cells release oxygen and nitrogen radicals to help kill the invaders and your finger gets red and inflamed as it tries to fight off any infection. That's your wonderful immune system in action. While you want free radicals to be mobilized when you cut your finger slicing that blasted tomato, you don't want these unstable and destructive compounds circulating inside your body over the long term.

Chronic, low-grade inflammation can produce a wide range of inflammatory proteins. These cause hormonal signaling to go haywire, and cause free radicals and pro-inflammatory compounds to flow freely at a low level...continually. Just like when you nick your finger and the inflammatory response begins, when those green beans hit your stomach, the immune system starts a chain reaction that prompts some of the body's cells to release histamine and other chemicals into the bloodstream. Because your body thinks that green beans are the enemy, it goes into high alert, thinking it's under attack. If you eat green beans regularly, your body will be in constant attack mode, which results in chronic inflammation—inflammation you may feel as joint pain, migraines, sinusitis, fatigue, depression, and even disease.

To control the histamine response, the body produces cortisol. You've no doubt heard the term cortisol—it's what we call the "stress hormone" because we secrete more of it when we're under psychological or physiological stress. When the body thinks it's under attack, it activates the "fight or flight" response, a physiological reaction designed to get your body ready to either fight the enemy or run away from it. The body pumps out cortisol to try to shut off the production of pro-inflammatory compounds and quickly release glucose, which your muscles can use for a surge of power.

If your body is constantly in a state of inflammation (which happens when you're downing green beans and other reactive foods right and left), your body will be constantly pumping out cortisol, sending signals to the body that it needs to be in a heightened defense mode, and store fat.

Can all that happen from some green beans? Absolutely.

Regulating Insulin—Vital for Your Success

There's a profound link between chronic inflammation and weight gain, leading to a vicious cycle. Fat cells generate chemical messengers which, over time, trigger a reaction for cells to stop responding to one of your body's critical messengers: insulin.

Insulin, which is produced by your pancreas, acts as a key allowing glucose—sugar—to get into your cells. Our cells use this sugar for energy.

However, chronic inflammation causes your cells' insulin receptors to become resistant, so your uptake of the sugars to your cells is not working effectively anymore. If the glucose can't get into your cells, it remains in your blood and starts to cause long-term damage, affecting your kidneys and liver and, left untreated, turns into diabetes. What my team and I find fascinating is that we see *any* reactive food can cause blood sugar levels to rise, not just sugars or carbs. Reactive to asparagus or turkey? Your blood sugar levels will go through the roof. More often than not, that excess glucose winds up stored as fat.

Even worse? Higher glucose levels will affect your thyroid, which is responsible for maintaining your metabolism. So you see how this can quickly go awry.

Penny, 33

Finding The Plan and introducing it to my family and friends has been life changing. I am a type 1 diabetic with hypothyroidism on an insulin pump. My husband and I were both exercising more than an hour a day before we started and had not been able to lose weight even though we eat very healthy. In the first week of becoming even more in tune with my body and food responses, I had to introduce apple, cranberry, and later mango juice as I reduced my basal insulin. In the first two weeks I kept backing off my basal insulin and barely used bolus insulin, even after having a cup of brown rice. I'm now eating three times as many carbs and taking one-third the amount of insulin. I've lost thirteen pounds and feel so much better. After two weeks my husband didn't have any pain in his shoulders or neck. Thank you for developing The Plan. I only wish that a nutritionist had introduced me to this concept when I was first diagnosed with diabetes twenty years ago.

Yeast—Maintain Your Balance

Before you do anything else, it's important to address a weight loss saboteur that prevents many people from taking off the weight: systemic yeast problems. Most people think that yeast is just a "female" problem, but everyone has yeast, and it can be found throughout our entire system.

The gut contains a delicate balance between friendly flora and yeast. Yeast colonies can multiply rapidly and overtake the friendly flora in response to diet, hormones, or environmental factors. Yeast feeds on sugar, so people who eat a lot of sugar are more prone to yeast overgrowth. Reactive foods can contribute to yeast overgrowth as can stress, birth control pills, medications, thyroid dysfunction, and exposure to radiation. Let's not forget hormonal changes—you know those mood swings and sugar and carb cravings you may have? You can blame yeast for part of that!

Regardless of the cause, yeast overgrowth can create digestive disturbances like bloating, gas, constipation, headache, sinus problems, brain fog, depression, and fatigue. While yeast organisms take over your intestinal flora, they produce acidic toxins, which slow down weight loss and affect your immune system.

To determine whether or not you have a yeast issue, try this simple test. Since yeast thrives on sugar and fermented foods, take a day to include in your menu wine or beer, balsamic vinegar, and chocolate. (I told you this wasn't any ordinary diet!) If you don't drink alcohol, just have the dessert and a heavy dose of a nice aged balsamic vinegar. Keep everything else the same as usual. The next day check your tongue in the mirror when you wake up. If it's coated white, yeast is an issue for you.

If so, don't panic! The best way to counteract a yeast overgrowth is through a course of high-quality probiotics. Probiotics are living organisms that are similar to the beneficial bacteria in your stomach that help restore the correct balance in your system. I like ReNew Life's (www.renewlife.com) Ultimate Flora Senior Formula 30 Billion—don't be put off by the name, I take it too when I need it! You can find it in the refrigerated section of health food stores and online. It's one that I find to work for just about everyone as it specifically has ten strains that are targeted for helping slowed digestion that comes with growing older.

Also don't fall into the trap of thinking that stronger is better when it comes to formulations! Probiotics with high-cell count can cause the yeast to die off too rapidly, which will cause an extreme detox with foggy thinking and severe mood swings. After about a week of probiotic treatment and eating your friendly foods you should have yeast under control.

Liselle, 56

I have been doing The Plan for ten days and I am thrilled with the results. I have lost twelve pounds and all my belly bloating and pain are gone. It is truly a miracle. I have been fighting systemic yeast for two years, which led me down a path of eating rice cakes, Greek yogurt, and Stevias. All of which I now know were hurting me. I was so confused and absolutely lost. I was not concerned with my weight but it was the bloating, headaches, and mood swings that were troubling me. I weighed 146 and now I am down to 134. The food is awesome. I will be on The Plan for life.

Goitrogens—Your Thyroid's Enemy

The thyroid is a major player when it comes to hormonal health since it stimulates and synchronizes all cellular function—primarily metabolism. Estrogen dominance and low testosterone have a lot to do with hampering the thyroid. Women can suffer from estrogen dominance as early as their twenties, but certainly it becomes much more routine after the age of thirty-five. Estrogen dominance is when progesterone drops

Is Your Thyroid Functioning at Its Peak?

Thyroid dysfunction can show up in many different ways. If you're experiencing any of these symptoms, you might have a thyroid issue:

- Depression
- Digestive problems
- Fatigue
- Feeling cold
- Hormonal imbalance
- Inability to lose weight
- Low sex drive
- Migraines
- Skin conditions

and estrogen is the dominant hormone (even if your estrogen level is low!). There is an increase in estrogen dominance during times of dramatic hormonal shifts, like post-partum and in perimenopause. Overexercising and diets low in animal protein can also lower the levels of free thyroid hormone in the body. Unfortunately, when your thyroid isn't functioning at its peak, it becomes much more difficult to lose weight.

Did You Know?

Did you know the thyroid only produces 1 teaspoon of thyroid hormone a year? Anything that affects the delicate balance of thyroid regulation can have dramatic effects on every function in our body.

A standard "healthy" diet usually includes foods known as *goitrogens*. Goitrogens are compounds found in certain foods that have been shown to interfere with thyroid function by blocking the enzymes which help produce thyroid hormones. (See the box on page 28 for a list of the most common goitrogenic foods.) Although many experts call these foods healthy, for those who are sensitive they are anything but. Certainly the more you rotate these foods the less of an effect they may have on your body. Note that cooking may deactivate goitrogens, especially for broccoli and kale. Juicing or eating these foods raw may increase their negative effect on the thyroid, which I'll explain in more detail in Chapter 3.

Before beginning the cleanse (which you'll find in Chapter 4), find out how your thyroid is functioning. For three days, keep a digital thermometer by your bed. When you wake up in the morning, place the thermometer under your armpit to get a read on your basal body temperature (BBT). Remember to keep still, as moving around will throw off the reading. A reading of 97.3°F or lower is an indication of a dysfunctional thyroid. I've found that about 85 percent of the women I work with and about 10 percent of younger men have thyroid issues. What's interesting is that as men age, they catch up with women. This number jumps to 40 percent in their forties, and by the time men are in their sixties they are almost neck and neck with women at 80 percent. The good news: When you identify the dysfunction before it gets to full-blown hyper- or hypothyroidism, it's easy to reverse.

But My Thyroid Tests Are Normal!

Thyroid tests use a very wide reference range and so what is normal for most people may not be "normal" for you. For example, let's say you are 5 feet 6 inches tall and female. The range for "normal weight" is 120 to 160 pounds. Now let's say you have been 123 pounds all your life and all of a sudden you step on the scale and you're 158. According to your doctor that would be normal. But it's not normal for *you*. Unfortunately most of us don't know our normal reference ranges for TSH, T4, and T3 (which are three hormones that are tested to determine whether or not your thyroid is working at the level it should) until we start testing them because we feel we may be hypo- or hyperthyroid! So we don't know what a normal range is for ourselves.

If you are lucky enough to have several years of thyroid info, see if numbers were in a consistent range when you felt well. That's probably *your* baseline.

Following The Plan and eating friendly foods, doing the proper amounts of exercise, and moderating stress will balance hormones and help with thyroid dysfunction. You will know when you are starting to heal your thyroid because your BBT will start to rise with right stimulus. If lamb or halibut is a friendly protein for your thyroid, your BBT will rise. If you are exercising at the right intensity for your body, your BBT will rise, too. Exercise too intensely or eat a goitrogen like spinach or strawberries? Your BBT will drop.

Are You Eating Goitrogenic Foods?

Here's a list of some of the most common goitrogenic foods that may be attacking your thyroid and affecting thyroid function. Note that cooking can deactivate the goitrogens, especially with broccoli and kale.

- Broccoli
- Broccoli rabe
- Brussels sprouts
- Cabbage
- Cauliflower
- Collards
- Horseradish
- Kale
- Millet
- Mustard
- Peaches
- Peanuts
- Pine nuts
- Radishes
- Raspberries
- Rutabaga
- Soybean and soy products, including tofu
- Spinach
- Strawberries
- Sweet potatoes
- Swiss chard
- Turnips
- Watercress

Marie, 31

I'm so thankful to have The Plan, it's changed my life so dramatically. When I first met Lyn-Genet she asked me for my current menu. I was so proud to share my turkey, Greek yogurt, and shrimp diet, thinking I was so on it. Guess what my most reactive list includes? Yup, all of the above. In combination with regular acupuncture, my migraines, which had become so bad I was an ER regular, are now gone! My life has changed completely and I'm an entirely new person, thanks to The Plan.

CHAPTER 3

Think It's Healthy? Think Again

Debunking the Myths that Sabotage Your Health

Experts talk every day about what's healthy and what's not. The media cries, "Eat more Greek yogurt!" "Stay away from gluten!" "Exercise harder!" And the public, trying desperately to get healthier, follows blindly. And yet even with all this effort, two-thirds of the adults in the United States are overweight or obese, according to the Centers for Disease Control and Prevention. You can't read your Facebook feed without hearing about a perfectly healthy friend who was diagnosed with some awful disease. You're trying to do all the right things. Why are you still cranky, stressed, tired, and feeling lousy?

I'll tell you why. When you hear something is "healthy," that statement is a mean average. So if something works for 70 percent of the population, the health and medical community thinks it's very effective. But many of us fall into the other 30 percent. And not just one time, but many times. It's easy to understand that the very things we're doing on a daily basis—things that pundits call healthy—are the very things that may be causing poor health and weight gain.

If you sign up for a diet program that allows you unlimited cauliflower (because, after all, it's a vegetable and all vegetables are healthy…), you can easily see how your well-intentioned efforts will backfire. Especially when you consider that cauliflower is 85 percent reactive!

I know I've said this before, but it's worth stressing again. The key to reducing inflammation, getting healthy, and losing weight is to find what works best for your body. Unfortunately, some of the most popular health and food trends today may not be healthy for you or your waistline. So if you feel like you aren't getting the results you deserve, it may be time to rethink a few things!

Rachel, 28

I want to say thank you. There are so many weight loss products and diets out there and The Plan is not about making money or tricking people into a crash diet that will be effective until you stop following its directions. If you commit, The Plan changes the way you eat and enjoy food so that it is a realistic lifestyle to adopt. Thank you for writing a book that gives people a plan to truly know their body and state of health. Knowing I can eat the foods I love (like cheese, chocolate, cereal, and chips) on a regular basis and still lose weight is sort of unbelievable. Not only that, but because of The Plan, I can still enjoy those foods that aren't as friendly as long as I work them into *my* plan and return to my friendly foods to give my inflamed body a break.

A million times, thank you. I am on my way to my goal weight and can't wait to get there. People in my life have noticed the changes I have made and it has inspired them to look at their health and food choices as well. My journey has even inspired a coworker, who started The Plan six days ago!

Juicing

Juicing is a hot trend today. Juicing fans state that your body absorbs more nutrients from juices than from whole fruit because you get the vitamins and minerals without the fiber that slows down how much food you can ingest. More nutrients must mean more health benefits, right?

However, when you remove all the pulpy fiber from fruit and carrots, you leave behind a heap of liquid sugar. Without fiber, the sugar is quickly absorbed and ready to spike your blood sugar and kick up some yeast. And if you're not juicing organic fruits, you're also rapidly absorbing a heap of pesticides. In contrast, the fiber in whole fruit slows down this rapid absorption of sugar and pesticides. Fiber gives the body time to try and fight the "bad guys" it sees in the pesticides. Speed it up by juicing the fruit and removing the fiber and our body just can't keep pace.

And if you're juicing for weight loss, you're not doing yourself any favors. Drinking juice all day doesn't teach you any new behaviors (it's certainly not sustainable), nor are you learning which foods really work for you. Unfortunately, long bouts of juicing can also damage your metabolism. You see, when you drastically reduce the number of calories you're taking in, the body goes into famine mode, holding on to every calorie it can by putting the brakes on your metabolism. The minute you put real food into your body, the weight comes flying back on because your metabolism has slowed to a screeching halt. So short-term weight loss in this case equals long-term metabolic knockout.

So many men and women cannot believe they can lose weight every day while still eating enough food to feel full and satisfied. Juicing can perpetuate this unhealthy cycle of "food fear" and keep you from learning to trust your body. Food is not the enemy, and I promise you can be healthier, leaner, and more vibrant when you eat your friendly foods and follow The Plan.

As I've mentioned in the previous chapter, many of the veggies and fruits that are popular for juicing—like spinach, kale, and strawberries—are goitrogenic. So, if your thyroid is already in a weakened state, all that raw spinach and kale is just going to weaken it further.

Is a juice every now and then potentially a healthy option? Absolutely! But regularly replacing meals with juices can have the opposite effect, causing damage to your short- and long-term health.

Allison, 46

I started The Plan because I was tired of being on a merry-go-round of trying to lose weight healthfully. I was a longtime vegetarian and when the weight wouldn't come off, I tried juicing. First one day a week, sometimes three days, and then I even did a weeklong fast. As soon as I ate real food, the weight would come back. I had a closet with three different sizes and was miserable. On top of it, I was chronically constipated, but the final straw was when my hair was falling out.

Then I heard about Lyn-Genet and The Plan and decided to buy the book. I did the cleanse and followed the book but after the first four days I couldn't lose one pound. Not

(Continued)

one! So I called and made an appointment and decided to work directly with Lyn-Genet. When she saw my diet she explained that I had primed my body to hold on to calories and we would have to retrain my body to know that food was coming in on a regular basis. Every time I would eat normally, my body would be afraid I'd go on another low-calorie diet and its job was to protect me from starvation so it would hold on to all the food I ate.

That made sense but really it was pretty frustrating. After almost four weeks I was ready to give up, but Lyn-Genet wouldn't let me. All of a sudden one day I woke up and lost weight! Then the next day, then the next. My body had finally let go and stopped being afraid I would keep starving myself. Frankly, I didn't think I could lose weight just by eating. But that's what happened. I can't believe what I did to my body for years. It makes me sad to think about it. Now I have great digestion, my hair's not falling out. I can be normal, go out with friends, and not be so obsessed. I know what works for me and I will never go back to being so unhealthfully "healthy."

Vegan

Vegans are definitely committed people! Not only do they shun all meat, fish, and poultry, they also don't eat any animal by-products such as eggs, honey, and dairy products. Vegan ideology is often focused not only on health, but on being kind to the planet and trying to leave as small a footprint as possible. I am down for that!

But because a vegan diet is already a limited diet, it can be hard to eat a healthy variety of foods—especially when you remember that you must rotate or react for best health. Vegan sources of proteins are pretty easy to break down in your twenties, but by the time you hit your forties and fifties, man can they be tough to digest! Beans, for example, cause gas for a reason. Gastrointestinal disturbance comes from foods that are taxing on your body to digest. While some beans like lentils and pinto beans are only 30 percent reactive, many other beans, like black beans, are 85 percent reactive. Even chickpeas, which are only 5 percent or so reactive, can start to pose problems if eaten too often. And the cellulose is really tough to break down. (Here's a tip though: You can buy hulled chickpeas, called chana dal, in most Indian markets.)

Any food consumed, no matter how healthy, can start to overload your organs and digestive system if you eat too much of it too often. Remember 70 percent of your immune system is in your gut, so for optimal health you need to have a wide variety of foods. This means you need to change up your foods on a regular basis so you don't build up food sensitivities. If your diet is limited to begin with, you may not have enough foods to put into the rotation.

On top of that, thyroid function diminishes as we age. A standard vegan diet is rich in goitrogenic foods such as tofu. Soy is a strong source of phytoestrogens, estrogen-like chemicals found in plant foods. Phytoestrogens latch on to the receptor sites on cells that are meant for estrogen, so they can skew estrogen levels and deactivate the thyroid. In addition, soy interferes with zinc absorption; zinc is a staple for immune function as well as prostate and digestive health.

I have found that for optimal health and weight most people's protein needs fall under these guidelines:

PROTEIN RANGES

	Women	*Men*
Breakfast	10 to 40 grams	15 to 60 grams
Lunch	15 to 25 grams	20 to 35 grams
Dinner	25 to 50 grams	40 to 70 grams

Any days you aren't meeting these requirements, you aren't giving yourself enough protein for healing your muscles, tissues, and cells. The body burns the most calories when it's repairing. Lowered protein consumption can lead to weight gain and poor health.

What about protein powders? These highly processed foods are usually very hard to digest, which as we know affects health and weight. You will definitely know if a protein powder doesn't work for you as you will start to bloat, have gas, and may notice decreased energy levels.

Have I had some vegans do The Plan successfully? Absolutely, and I'm thrilled they found a way to find the foods that worked for them and maintain their ideals. But some have not. How have we dealt with this at The Plan? It can be very hard to go through your diet and your beliefs and find that they're not working for your body. We have a simple saying at the office: Being kind to the earth starts with yourself first. If being vegan works for you, then totally rock it! But if it doesn't, then try to listen to your body and take care of yourself. Things have a wonderful way of working out where you can still leave a small footprint and make clean, conscious choices.

Supplements for Vegans

Garden of Life probiotics and Premier Research probiotics are two brands highly recommended by my vegan Planners. Liquid B12 is very easy to absorb and essential for vegans as the diet is naturally low in B12, which is essential for absorption of iron and thyroid health and is necessary for a healthy nervous system. Vegans can also have a tendency toward anemia because it can be hard to get sufficient iron from plant foods alone. Many iron supplements cause constipation, but two brands I like are Ferrochel (non-binding), which is a capsule, and Floradix, which is liquid. A great tip for vegan kids? The liquid is really easy to add to soups and pancake mixes if your kids are vegan and low in iron!

Raw Foods

Raw food advocates state that plant foods in their most natural state—uncooked and unprocessed—are the most wholesome for the body. Raw foodists, as they're called, do not cook with temperatures over about 115°F.

I have found that as we age a total raw food diet is just too hard on digestion for many. If you impair digestion, you impede weight loss and immune function. Some raw fruits and veggies are essential, but too much of a good thing is, well, never good!

In traditional Chinese medicine, the stomach and spleen use energy to "cook" our food. You've no doubt heard the word *chi*, life's energy force, in Chinese medicine. One of the goals in Chinese medicine is for the body to work together to be in balance and harmony. When the spleen and stomach are using up their chi to heat up and digest food, it throws the body out of balance. In other words, when you overtax one organ—in this case the stomach or spleen—it will start to affect all the other organs, creating a negative domino effect. Your chi, your life force, will in effect become depleted.

From a Western point of view, vegetables are loaded with cellulose, an organic compound that provides structure and strength to the cell walls of plants and provides us with fiber. Although some animals can digest cellulose incredibly well, it's very problematic for many humans, so it can cause gas and bloating. For those with weakened digestion, it can also lead to inflammation. Many vegetables actually have more bioavailable nutrients when they are cooked, like carrots, tomatoes, and green leafy vegetables. I also talked earlier about how many vegetables are goitrogenic in their raw state, so raw foodists may be missing out on so many of the nutritional benefits of vegetables, and are damaging their thyroid.

Does cooking kill live enzymes in foods? Yes. Can most people tolerate small amounts of raw food without hampering digestion? Absolutely! Why not have the best of both worlds and eat small amounts of raw vegetables to get the live enzymes, plus cooked vegetables to aid digestion? In Chapter 7, Salads and Soups, we will discuss further some optimal ratios of cooked to raw foods.

Gluten Free

About 30 percent of Americans are staying away from gluten. I will admit, gluten is the toughest part of bread to digest, so if you're eating bagels day after day (bagels, pasta, and pizza dough have extra gluten added to them), you will most likely build up a gluten intolerance. Many Plan followers who thought they were reactive to wheat found that after a three-day cleanse, they tolerated wheat just fine in moderation. I find that if you do well on bread, you will keep doing well on bread and wheat products if you have them two to three times a week. The key is always try to give your body a break, and keep those friendly foods in rotation.

Whether you want to stay gluten free or are diagnosed with celiac disease, gluten-free products can be problematic themselves. The alternate grains used to make these products are often reactive. Two big players in gluten-free bread are tapioca starch and potato starch. Tapioca rates a 94 out of a possible 100 on the glycemic index (GI), which is a method of measuring how a food affects insulin and blood sugar levels. The higher the GI number, the more it has a negative effect. Consumption of high-glycemic foods results in increase of blood glucose levels, which increases insulin production and sets us up for some serious problems. Potato starch isn't any better as it has been linked to various disorders such as arthritis, eczema, psoriasis, and fibromyalgia.

Quinoa and teff, two other big gluten alternatives, are also both highly inflammatory. And for a good reason. Please consider this before jumping on the latest ancient grain bandwagon. The body is pretty amazing in its streamlining operations. If a grain isn't around for a few thousand years, the body will often lose the enzymes to break it down. Teff is from Ethiopia and quinoa is from the Andes. If you are from either of these regions, you have a much better chance of digesting these grains, but if not, you might have to wait a few thousand more years before your body is able to digest them. If you do use quinoa, make sure to rinse it thoroughly; the saponins in quinoa can cause eye and respiratory issues as well as gastrointestinal distress.

Xanthan gum, a plant-based thickening and stabilizing agent often added to products in place of gluten, is high in purines, natural substances found in all of the body's cells. When cells die and get recycled, the purines in their genetic material also get broken down and they turn into uric acid, which can aggravate pain and inflammation. This is especially noted for people with gout.

Corn is 90 to 95 percent reactive with my clients and it is often genetically modified. Even if you buy organic corn, GMO may still be a problem. Experts fear that cross-pollination has already begun with GMO corn, as the pollen grains are among the largest and heaviest of wind-pollinated plants. I often see clients gain a pound from the simple pleasure of a summer corn on the cob.

So what does this mean if you can't tolerate gluten? That you shouldn't have any sort of bread at all? That's not the purpose of this information. Really, I'm not here to torture you! What I do want you to know is that if you find your body is not responding the way it should, perhaps the fact that you're eating gluten free is actually the problem. Try to avoid those gluten-free products for a few days to give your body a chance to rest and decrease inflammatory response.

For our gluten-free and paleo friends, I have found that rice flour, coconut flour, and almond flour are the most easily digested. Please avoid brown rice flour products as the arsenic content is much higher. It's also important to remember that just because something is proinflammatory for a certain population it does not mean it's going to be a problem for you. Just listen to your body—it will always tell you everything you need to know.

Overexercising

Yes, yes, I know what you're thinking. How can you exercise too much? It's true. Over-training can slow weight loss and repair. Remember what I've said about how calories don't matter? That doesn't apply just to eating calories; it applies to burning them as well.

Studies are consistently showing that you can have the same amount of weight loss in a sixty-minute workout as a twenty- to thirty-minute workout. Experience with thou-sands of clients has shown us at The Plan that overtraining not only impedes weight loss but can also cause weight gain!

Cindy, 44

Prior to discovering The Plan, I struggled with weight loss and I mean struggled. I tried all the diets and different ways of eating. I exercised like crazy, and I mean crazy! I did a sprint distance triathlon and ran a half marathon and all to no avail. I didn't even lose a pound while training for those events. Not a pound! I did P90X workouts and took Spinning classes...it didn't help with weight loss. I found The Plan and had some struggles figuring out how this body worked, but The Plan made perfect sense so I contacted and worked with Lyn-Genet. Things started making some sense, but weight loss was still slow, so Lyn suggested we add some exercise. After I reined in my "don't dare ask me to exercise because that doesn't work for me" attitude I listened to what she had to say. I started with seven to eight minutes (just to appease Lyn) every other day, and much to my skeptical eye the weight loss increased. I was "wowed"! We slowly, and I mean slowly, increased the time I spent exercising, I've never spent more than thirty minutes working out since I started The Plan. I don't miss the long, hard workouts I used to do and now relish the fact that I've lost weight, almost thirty pounds, without long workouts.

I am so thankful for finding The Plan. I'm forty-four years old and have never looked or felt better! Thanks, Lyn-Genet!

In addition to the weight gain, we see a corresponding decrease in basal body temperature (BBT) and increased high blood pressure. With skewed BBT, we see worsening PMS, infertility, menopausal difficulties, depression, digestive issues—you name it. As soon as I have my clients decrease their exercise to what works for their bodies, we see hormones, body, and mood rebalance.

Here's what we've found at The Plan, after compiling data from thousands of clients over eight years:

- Women (and men over the age of forty) who exercise five to six days a week lose 25 percent less weight than those who exercise three to four times a week.
- Exercising for more than thirty to forty-five minutes (depending on the exercise—read on for more details) slows weight loss or causes weight gain.
- The biggest culprits are boot camp, CrossFit-style classes, Bikram yoga, and Spinning.

While people may be tempted to say that this weight gain could be attributed to building muscle, we have found that the days where there is weight gain from exercise there is also a corresponding aggravation of people's health issues: For instance, blood pressure and blood sugar levels will rise as BBT drops. This indicates the exercise is affecting much more than hypertrophy and muscle repair and is actually causing an inflammatory response in the body.

Exercise and Cortisol

Overexercising puts stress on your body. If you're exercising too hard, your body gets the message that it needs to hold on to more calories to keep up with the energetic demands you're putting on it. It doesn't know how much energy you're going to need, so it adapts to the energy requirements you're programming into it and holds on to more and more calories for potential future survival. Remember, your body's goal is to keep you alive, and when you program it to think that it always needs a reserve to live off, it's going to hold on to that fat for dear life!

Exercising too intensely can increase oxidative stress, which your body has a harder time dealing with as you get older. The increase in free radicals can do a lot of damage to your cell walls and this is how we set ourselves up for heart disease and diseases like cancer.

In addition, overexercising will increase cortisol levels, which increases insulin output and encourages fat storage. In fact, cortisol can *suppress* metabolic activity to preserve energy. The increase in cortisol can deplete progesterone or testosterone levels, another reason for weight gain and thyroid dysfunction. And research has shown that when you exercise for more than half an hour, your appetite increases, thus often offsetting the metabolic boost and calorie-burning activity.

So in the end, you're creating a calorie surplus, not a deficit. You already know that heightened cortisol levels start to skew hormone and endocrine function....I should see a lightbulb going off now. Is it any wonder that you are having a hard time losing weight with all the exercise you are doing?

The *Need* to Exercise

Many of my clients tell me they have to exercise or they'll kill someone. But I think this is one of those chicken/egg things. When you exercise you boost serotonin, but when you go too far you're heightening those cortisol levels. So what winds up happening is your fuse is a little bit shorter the next day and you're more stressed out. So you feel that urge to work out, to boost the serotonin levels again. You go for your run, you get that short-term boost of serotonin so you feel really good, but you also get the extra production of cortisol so once again, your fuse is shorter the next day. Oh, and by the way, you're gaining weight.

We find that many people who feel that they need to exercise to deal with anxiety, anger, or stress actually discover that they are less stressed when they start following our guidelines. They also have more time to spend relaxing with friends and family as well as finding hobbies that decrease their stress.

So, Should You Skip Exercise Altogether?

Absolutely not. I'm not against all exercise. I know it's crucial for cardiovascular health, stress reduction, mood elevation, bone density, and a sense of well-being and confidence. In my early thirties I was a maniac, running fifty miles a week, every single week, *and* in the gym six days a week. But here I am at almost fifty, I've had a child, and I only exercise thirty minutes, three to four times a week; my body fat is exactly the same as it was, *plus* I weigh five pounds less. "Smarter, not harder" should be the mantra for most of us.

If you're training for a sport or competition, that's one thing. But if you're exercising intensely to burn calories and lose weight, it's probably not going to do what you want as you get older. The body burns the most energy when it's doing repair, not when it's exercising. If you look at the caloric expenditure when you're exercising, it can be nominal. But when you're sleeping and doing deep repair, you can lose three pounds!

So, what does that mean for you? In order to avoid health and weight frustrations, we encourage our clients to "test" their favorite exercise as a health variable to see exactly how it affects their bodies. Try a different frequency, different intensity, a different duration, and see how your body reacts. We've found that people who exercised every other day have the best results for weight loss. I recommend either thirty minutes of weight training or weight training and cardio mixed in with some yoga and body weighted exercises.

I'm not a big fan of cardio for an extended period of time as you age. That's because exercise tends to be proinflammatory and increase oxidative stress when it is done for an extended period of time with no decrease in heart rate. When we're younger we have a defense system known as super oxide dismutase (SOD) that can vanquish free radicals, but as we get older, SOD doesn't work as well as it used to. Simply taking breaks and allowing your heart rate to decrease to a normal resting level can make all the difference! Not just that, but doing intervals—when you go hard for a few minutes and then pull back and recover for a few minutes—can be far more efficient than long, steady activity.

Where does this leave you? Well, it's always about finding your own path. Some people are blessed with the genes to be more athletic with less stress on their bodies. Planners have included Ironmen, triathletes, and marathoners, and this intensity may be the *best* thing for you. But if exercise is leaving you feeling like the effort you are putting in isn't paying off with better weight and health, it's time for a new plan.

The Three-Day Cleanse

I've told you already that this cookbook is full of recipes that are not just easy to prepare, but friendly for the whole family. That's mainly because they're full of foods that we've found to be almost universally low inflammatory, have a healing effect, and promote weight loss.

If you've already done The Plan from my first book, you know the healing power of a cleanse. And even if you're already doing The Plan, you may want to do a refresher cleanse.

If you're new to my program, then this cleanse is absolutely essential for you. Why? You've been eating lots of foods that you've been told are healthy, and we've already discussed why these foods may not work for you at all. So the cleanse is going to clear your body of that inflammation it's been holding on to for all these years, and bring it back to the place it wants to be—a natural state of homeostasis.

Sophia, 61

My husband is diabetic and he has not taken any meds for the past few years. Within three days of starting the cleanse, his blood sugar reading went from 287 to 151! I am also following The Plan, as are three of our daughters, and we are all feeling wonderful! Thanks so much!

Notes about Animal Protein

Most proteins, if they can be eaten rare, should be. Proteins and fats can be very sensitive to heat and they start to change their molecular structure and become more inflammatory when overcooked. So beef carpaccio—super friendly! Beef stew—maybe not as much. What we have also found with animal proteins is that the higher omega-3 contents are especially sensitive to heat. So when possible, try to have those free-range meats cooked as rare as possible. This is also why salmon sashimi digests so well, while cooked salmon is 85 percent reactive!

Throughout your life, the body wants to renew and repair. That's what it's designed to do. But when we fill it with foods that are reactive, the body's energy is diverted from a state of homeostasis to the most immediate task at hand—attacking the reactive food it perceives as the enemy—and veers off its intended course. This causes an inflammatory response that can last up to seventy-two hours. But when we give it a little nudge by detoxing, it gets right back onto the path of self-healing. We also instinctively start to crave healthier foods. So it's a win-win situation.

So, before you dive headfirst into the wonderful recipes in this book, let's wipe the slate clean in your body. Not only will that rid you of the inflammation that's been causing you trouble, it will also sensitize your palate. The cleanse will rid your diet of the excess salt (rampant in processed foods), which will attune your taste buds to all the other flavors you've been missing. I have clients tell me all the time that they never realized how delicious food was—or how salty restaurant food is—until after they'd done the cleanse. Excess sodium raises blood pressure, increases risk of cardiovascular disease, causes water retention, creates sugar cravings, and exacerbates reactive response to an inflammatory food. Reducing its presence in your system sets you up for better success with the foods you'll be making later in the book.

Ready to start the cleanse and get back on the path to health? Let's do it!

CHAPTER 4

The Cleanse

Repair and Rejuvenate

I have been using a food-based cleanse for over twenty-five years and I can't think of a faster way to kick-start healing and amazing weight loss. The cleanse is designed to keep you full, all while allowing the body to take a break from digesting food that takes more energy to break down. Most people like to shop on Saturday, prep on Sunday, and start their cleanse on a Monday, but of course you should do what works best for *you*.

These three days are a nutritional powerhouse chock-full of healing foods. The meals and days are also chemically balanced, so it's important that even if you're full you have a little of each dish. Full? On a cleanse? Oh yes, most people aren't used to having each of their meals nutrient dense and full of protein, good fats, and fiber. Every meal in the cleanse has this balance, so you should be wonderfully full.

For the next three days you will be consuming anywhere from 80 to 100-plus grams of vegetarian protein to aid repair. Remember, your body burns a lot of calories when it's repairing. In addition, higher protein diets seem to keep hormones like ghrelin, which spike appetite, at bay. The cleanse is also rich in fiber that helps to keep you full (and your intestines happy!).

Fiber has many amazing properties. Fiber:

- reduces cholesterol.
- promotes bowel regularity.

- reduces cardiovascular disease.
- prevents colon cancer.
- prevents constipation.
- reduces diabetes.
- helps to heal diverticulitis.

What If I Have Diverticulosis?

Each person's tolerance to fiber is different. In America, our diet is typically low in fiber and many people are still being informed that if they have diverticulosis they need to have a diet low in fiber. This is actually not true; it is only through higher fiber diets that your body will heal. You should however avoid high fiber if you are in the active state of diverticulosis, which is called diverticulitis. Because each person's tolerance to fiber is different, I recommend that you only do the cleanse under the guidance of a Plan nutritionist. We usually start you off with a modified diet to slowly reintroduce fiber so you won't have a flare-up, and of course you should always consult with your health care provider before embarking on any major dietary change.

The cleanse will also reset your palate, which has been overloaded with salt and sugar. Each time a new food is introduced it's like a taste symphony. Day Two, rice for dinner? Amazing. Day Three with chicken? You've never tasted anything more delicious. When coffee, cheese, wine, and chocolate are introduced as part of your regimen right after the cleanse, it's like the angels are singing! What's really amazing though is that when "normal" foods are introduced, especially prepared foods, you will be shocked at how salty and full of chemicals so many foods you consumed were!

Felicia, 28

I made it through the cleanse and I couldn't wait to dive into dessert after the cleanse. I had some of my favorite chocolate pudding as soon as I could. I could not believe how disgusting it tasted; it just tasted like chocolate chemicals. I used to eat this pudding every day as my treat! I couldn't believe that just a few days could change the way I felt about foods so quickly.

In the rest of the book, the recipes introduced are thyroid friendly and contain the foods we've found to be the lowest-inflammatory foods. There are recipes for everyone in this book: health enthusiasts, gluten-free devotees, vegetarians, vegans, and paleo enthusiasts. Following The Plan protein guidelines (see page 35) will help you reach your health and weight goals quicker, and following hydration rules (see page 49) will up your energy levels, help to conquer constipation, and make your skin glow.

If you haven't done the twenty days just yet and you just want to do the cleanse and enjoy the recipes, that's fine! Try MSM, probiotics, and SAM-e on an as-needed basis, see how you feel after each meal, and listen to your body, and you are on your way to becoming a seasoned Planner!

Supplements: A Refresher

As I explained in Chapter 2, I'm not a huge fan of taking supplements indefinitely, but they can help as needed or for short periods of time. Here's a refresher on my favorites.

SAM-e: Take to mitigate cortisol/stress response and bring hormones back in balance. Aids weight loss which has been hampered by stress. Do not take daily—only on an as-needed basis. Planners find that 600 milligrams in the morning works best.

Probiotics: Take when yeast is active to restore immune functioning, gastrointestinal balance, and hormonal balance. Do not take daily, only when yeast is active or when you have a reaction to a food. Best taken in the morning.

MSM: Take to restore mucosal strength; for instance, to help with asthma, GERD (gastroesophageal reflux disease), or sinusitis, or with gastrointestinal issues like chronic constipation, Crohn's, colitis, IBS (irritable bowel syndrome), leaky gut, etc. Therapeutic dose is traditionally for six weeks and then use is discontinued. Dose ranges from 3,000 to 6,000 milligrams daily, taken all at once.

Liquid B12 and Maine Coast Sea Seasonings or kelp: Take only if BBT is consistently below 96.3. Take until BBT boosts to high 96/97 to restore thyroid function and hormonal balance.

The Cleanse

Cleansing the digestive system is a practice that dates back to ancient times. From Ayurvedic medicine to Zen Buddhism, nearly every culture and religion throughout the centuries recognized the benefit of detoxifying the body through a cleanse, a fast, or abstinence from certain foods to establish better digestive health and focus intention and purpose.

We have helpful hints on our website www.lyngenet.com to prep the food as quickly as possible, and if you're comfortable in the kitchen you can make the food for all three days in less than an hour and a half. To make things easier and keep costs down, we take leftovers from most dinners and use them for lunch the next day. This means less work and less money spent. Rest assured, while you are cooking most of your meals, I want it to be as easy as possible.

What You Need to Know

For these next three days, you'll be giving your body a break from the difficult task of digesting reactive and processed foods, allowing it to reset and return to its natural state. Think of this time as a present to yourself. Gentle stretches, saunas or warm baths, gentle walks, and massages will aid your body's healing and help you feel good. Family members and friends often like to do the cleanse together to share stories, help each other cook, and cheer on each other each day.

In the morning of each day of the cleanse, please remember to:

1. **Weigh yourself.** This is hard for many people, but I can't say it enough—the scale is your best friend. It is going to end the mystery of why you gain weight and how to lose weight. Weight is just data. It's a number that reflects information from the prior day's stimulus of food, water, stress, and exercise.
2. **Drink water with lemon.** After you weigh yourself, please drink sixteen ounces of fresh water with lemon juice. Add as much lemon juice as you like. I like it pretty lemony so I use bottled Santa Cruz Organic lemon juice and just squeeze a little fresh lemon on top for fresh vitamin C. Many people also find lemon juice helpful to get extra water down, so feel free to have a couple of pints of lemon

water during the day if you'd like. Just be careful to brush your teeth throughout the day as too much lemon can affect tooth enamel.

In addition to the lemon water, I recommend that you take a liver detox herb like milk thistle or dandelion (both of which you can take as a capsule). If pills aren't your thing have some dandelion tea an hour after breakfast.

The liver gets a lot of love on The Plan, and there's a reason for that. It's responsible for over five hundred functions, including metabolism and hormonal control. Each day you start your morning with lemon juice and water to aid liver function and then you use dandelion tea or a liver cleanser for even more support for the full three days of the cleanse (and full twenty days if you're embarking on the program outlined in *The Plan*). After that you can take a break from these. Remember we always want to rotate everything!

Each morning of the cleanse begins with Flax Granola (page 68). Flaxseeds are rich in protein, fiber, omega-3s, and calcium. Flax granola is pretty awesome. The recipe calls for whole flaxseeds soaked overnight so they can release mucilage. I like to compare mucilage to the scrubby bubbles—they not only clean your intestines but get in the nooks and crannies so you don't wind up with inflamed intestines and diverticulitis! However, I want to make sure you understand flax is not a laxative and you won't have to run to the bathroom, so no fear there! It just aids output and frequency. If constipation has been a problem for you, flax granola will be your best friend.

After the first week of Planning, please limit the flax granola to twice a week for maximum health benefits. Remember rotate or react is The Plan motto, and I'll be giving you plenty of other great, tasty, breakfast recipes later in the book!

Water—The Pint Method

It's crucial to drink water based on your mass and hydration needs. Water consumption is based on your weight; you should drink approximately half your body weight in ounces every day. Skimping on even one glass will show up on the scale. Why? Your body needs water to carry out every one of its metabolic and cellular functions.

When you don't drink enough water, you're basically telling the body it's okay to not repair the heart, liver, and lungs and that instead it should divert a lot of energy extracting water from all the foods you're eating and liquids you're drinking. Water is then held in your tissues as a reservoir so you have enough water for daily functioning in an all-too-common phenomenon we know as "water weight." When you drink appropriate amounts of water, your body says, "Hey all that water I was holding on to, I can let go of that," and then you lose water weight! I have so many people say that the week prior to starting their Plan they started hydrating and lost anywhere from five to seven pounds.

Make sure to get your water in between meals, not during meals, as drinking during meals can impair digestion. If you can, leave a forty-five-minute window before and after each meal. Finish all your water by dinner and do not consume *any* after dinner. I know so many of us think that more is better, but this is definitely not the case with water. Consuming too much water will cause water retention and start to stress kidney function.

Now here's the deal. I'm sure if you liked water you would drink enough. But you're probably like most people and drink much less than you should. So, here's my thought on hydration: If you don't like water don't sip it all day, knock it back all at once in a pint glass! For example, if you're 200 pounds, you need to drink six pints throughout the day. First thing in the morning I want you to have one pint with your lemon juice. That means just programming five more pints through the day. Schedule one at 9 a.m., one at 12 noon, one at 2 p.m., 5 p.m., and 7 p.m., and you are done for the day.

Even better news? When you drink a pint all at once your body takes what it needs and excretes the rest, so you can time your bathroom breaks. I actually devised this method thanks to schoolteachers, bless their hearts! Every teacher I worked with was chronically dehydrated because they couldn't leave the classroom to go to the bathroom. With the pint method they were able to meet their hydration needs, lose weight, and keep their students from staging a coup!

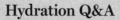

Hydration Q&A

What else can I drink besides water?

Most herbal teas, like peppermint tea, chamomile tea, white tea, and rooibos teas, are all fine to have included as part of your water intake. You may also have green or black tea, but I would limit those to sixteen ounces daily because of their acidity. I don't recommend teas that contain licorice or chicory without testing—they could be reactive.

Does coffee count as part of my water intake when I include it after the cleanse?

No, coffee doesn't count toward your daily water total. You do not need to include extra water for drinking up to twelve ounces of coffee, which is the limit on The Plan.

Should I add extra water for when I drink wine and when is it best to have wine?

After the three-day cleanse, red wine with dinner is great to lower cortisol levels and aid digestion. It's best to add an extra four ounces of water to your daily intake before dinner for every glass of wine you have. Please do not add water after dinner and of course if you don't wish to drink wine, don't!

When do I need to stop drinking water?

While eating late is fine for some people, I find that for optimal digestion it's critical to not to drink water with or after dinner and at least three to four hours before bed.

How do I adjust my water intake for exercise?

A good rule of thumb is to add eight ounces for every thirty minutes of exercise. You may drink less or more according to thirst.

How do I adjust water intake for hot weather?

In hot weather, make adjustments to your water intake the way you would based on your exercise (one or two additional glasses depending upon the severity of the heat, how much time you spend outdoors, etc.). This is especially important for those of you who get migraines, because heat can dehydrate you and trigger migraines. Staying out in the heat too long can start to cause your body to overheat and impair your lymphatic system. We see this especially when people garden outdoors for hours. It is best to take breaks from the heat by going inside and cooling off every thirty minutes if possible. You may notice weight stabilization the next day.

General Guidelines for the Cleanse

While doing your cleanse, please remember the following:

- Follow the menus exactly. Do not make substitutions or changes.
- Salad dressing for the cleanse should consist of lemon juice, extra virgin olive oil (EVO), and herbs of choice (I like dill, parsley, and oregano). Avoid vinegar so you can let the yeast population decrease. You may also use the Lime Agave Vinaigrette (page 148).
- Do not consume coffee during the cleanse. If you are concerned about a caffeine headache, you may have black tea with lemon. Green tea is acceptable, but please note it may aggravate acid reflux more than black tea. All teas count toward your water intake. Please limit caffeinated teas to sixteen ounces a day and please do not use with sweetener during the cleanse. Teas with Stevia may cause weight stabilization instead of weight loss, because the processing of stevia leaf can contain as many as forty known toxins such as acetone and ethanol.

Carly, 44

My kids are already benefiting from my cleanse. It's easy to feed my family with what I've made. They ate up the rice, carrots, and blueberries. I just added a simple protein for them and dinner is done. My four-year-old loves the blueberry compote and my teenager snacks on the flax granola like it's popcorn!

The Plan for Day One

Note: There are no portions for lunch and dinner. Eat until you are full and please make sure to have part of each recommended dish. Please remember to include EVO, lemon juice, and herbs of choice at lunch as your salad dressing.

UPON AWAKENING

Weigh yourself.

Start your day with 16 ounces warm lemon juice and water and a liver cleanser. All waters and teas count toward your water intake.

BREAKFAST

For women: 1 cup Flax Granola (page 68) with ½ pear
For men: 1½ cups Flax Granola (page 68) with 1 pear
Silk coconut milk or Rice Dream—any amount up to 12 ounces
OR
For women: 2 cups Warm Raisin Flax Cereal (page 70) with ½ pear
For men: 3 to 4 cups Warm Raisin Flax Cereal (page 70) with 1 pear

LUNCH

Carrot Ginger Soup (page 101) with chia seeds or sunflower seeds
Steamed broccoli with lemon juice and EVO
Baby romaine with ½ pear and pumpkin seeds

SNACK

1 medium apple

DINNER

Kale in Spicy Coco Sauce (page 156)
Carrot Beet Salad (page 96) with pumpkin seeds

Note: If you are above your set weight you should lose at least 1 pound. People have lost as much as 9 pounds on Day One! If you don't lose weight, organs of elimination may be overloaded and weight loss should resume on Day Two.

The Plan for Day Two

Note: There are no portions for lunch and dinner. Eat until you are full and please make sure to have part of each recommended dish. Please remember to include EVO, lemon juice, and herbs of choice at lunch as your salad dressing.

Day Two incorporates your first test, which is almonds. Please make sure to choose raw unsalted almonds. Roasted nuts, while delicious, are higher in reactivity unless you roast them yourself at a low temperature and consume within a week or two of eating. You can find a recipe for Roasted Nuts on page 115.

UPON AWAKENING

Weigh yourself.

Start your day with 16 ounces warm lemon juice and water and a liver cleanser. All waters and teas count toward your water intake.

Note: if you feel the detox is a little intense, you can move the rice from dinner to lunch. Rice will slow the detox down.

BREAKFAST

For women: 1 cup Flax Granola (page 68) with ½ pear

For men: 1½ cups Flax Granola (page 68) with 1 pear

Silk coconut milk or Rice Dream—any amount up to 12 ounces

LUNCH

Carrot Ginger Soup (page 101) with pumpkin seeds

Baby romaine with radicchio, apple, and raw sunflower seeds

SNACK

For women: 1 apple with 8 raw almonds

For men: 1 apple with 16 to 18 raw almonds

DINNER

For women: leftover Kale in Spicy Coco Sauce, and 1 cup Indian "Lentils" with Basmati Rice (page 156) with pumpkin seeds

For men: leftover Kale in Spicy Coco Sauce, and 1½ to 2 cups Indian "Lentils" with Basmati Rice (page 156) with pumpkin seeds

Baby Romaine with Carrot Beet Salad (page 96) with sunflower seeds

Note: If you are not at your set weight, you should lose at least 1 pound. If you do not, you are reactive to almonds. Please cut them out going forward. This is especially common in people who have been overeating almonds. You may just need to lay off almond usage for 3 months and then retest. Remember that many gluten-free and paleo products use almonds and almond flour and you may have built up an almond sensitivity.

The Plan for Day Three

Chicken is the least reactive protein, closely followed by lamb. It is a wonderful, low-cost protein and a large part of many people's diets. Because it is such a mainstay for so many people, and may be eaten a bit too often, you want to make sure it works for you. If you choose to not test chicken and would like to test another low-reactive animal protein you can test lamb, beef, flounder, or sashimi.

UPON AWAKENING

Weigh yourself.

Start your day with 16 ounces warm lemon juice and water and a liver cleanser. All waters and teas count toward your water intake.

BREAKFAST

For women: 1 cup Flax Granola (page 68) with ½ pear

For men: 1½ cups Flax Granola (page 68) with 1 pear

Silk coconut milk or Rice Dream—any amount up to 12 ounces

Or

For women: 2 cups Warm Raisin Flax Cereal (page 70) with ½ pear

For men: 3 to 4 cups Warm Raisin Flax Cereal (page 70) with 1 pear

LUNCH

Baby romaine with carrots, and pumpkin seeds

Cream of Broccoli Soup (page 103)

SNACK

For women: 12 raw almonds or ½ apple (if reactive to almonds)

For men: 18 raw almonds or 1 apple (if reactive to almonds)

DINNER

For women: 2 to 3 ounces of Chicken with Italian Herbs and Orange Zest (page 169), Radicchio and Pomegranate Salad (page 96), Roasted Vegetables (page 126)

For men: 4 ounces of Chicken with Italian Herbs and Orange Zest (page 169), Radicchio and Pomegranate salad (page 96), Roasted Vegetables (page 126)

Spice It Up!

Not only can you include these seasonings whenever you can, I encourage them. They are good for the digestion and help ease inflammation. You can also try most salt-free blends as long as they don't have paprika or licorice.

- Basil
- Black pepper
- Cardamom
- Cayenne
- Cinnamon
- Cumin
- Ground ginger
- Maine Coast Sea Seasonings (kelp or dulse varieties)
- Rosemary
- Turmeric
- Organic lemon, lime, or orange zest
- Garlic
- Onion
- Dill
- Parsley
- Sage
- Mint
- Oregano
- Thyme

Cleanse Fallout

Even though this is a food-based detox, it's still a detox and you may experience some unpleasant symptoms such as headaches and fatigue. It's better to get this stuff out now, rather than let it keep piling up in your system! What you are experiencing is decades of toxins being released from your system. In fact, people are surprised the second time they do the cleanse because there is often no discomfort or fatigue at all. Hang in there! These kinds of symptoms are perfectly normal, and thankfully, they usually pass within the first twenty-four to forty-eight hours.

I also recommend that you not work out during the cleanse. For the next three days, your body's energy needs to be funneled toward repair. If you work out during this time, you'll divert energy to exercise and muscle repair, leaving less for renewing vital organs.

You may also find that you want to sleep. A lot. This is great because sleep is the time your body repairs most. So try to set aside some time so you can go to bed early and let your body heal itself. You won't believe how good you will feel. Many people have also noted that this is a time when they process emotions that have been pent-up for years. Remember the cleanse is about not just shedding pounds, but making new and healthier paths in your life.

Following are some other helpful hints to get you through the worst of it. If you have:

- **A headache**: Double-strength peppermint tea works wonders. If you must take a pain reliever, choose acetaminophen over ibuprofen. Ibuprofen can cause water retention. Excedrin Migraine works well for intense headaches.
- **Fatigue, lethargy, or weakness**: Rest as much as possible—your body needs it. It's trying to repair and that takes a lot of work.
- **Light-headedness or muscle cramps**: Make sure you're drinking enough water and consuming enough fats (don't skimp on the seeds or EVO!). Emergen-C may help but can cause water retention.
- **Irritability**: Studies have shown that SAM-e is an effective liver cleanser and aids the uptake of dopamine, norepinephrine, and serotonin, which decreases depression and anxiety.
- **Flu-like symptoms**: Try a hot bath with Epsom salts and baking soda.
- **A coated, pasty tongue**: This is a sign of a systemic yeast overgrowth dying off. A few days of a probiotic can help restore gastrointestinal balance.
- **Constipation, diarrhea, or gas**: Try ginger, peppermint, or chamomile tea. Many people's bodies are so used to having coffee-initiated peristalsis that when

they stop drinking coffee, their bowel movements stop as well. Do not take any laxatives, even "natural" ones, as they create dependency. Better to try and let your body take a few days off from artificial stimulus and figure out how to work on its own again.

- **Mood swings:** Meditation can help with the range of emotions you may experience during the cleanse.
- **General blahs:** Hot showers can be very helpful. Make the water as hot as you can stand it and scrub the skin well. This will help to eliminate toxins through the skin. Saunas, massage, and light stretching are also all wonderful to assist your body in releasing toxins.

Colette, 34

During the cleanse I doubled the recipes to share with my husband and kids if they were feeling brave. (Might not have needed to double. Wow that's a lot of food!) My nine-year-old boy and his buddy walked in and said, "What are you cooking? Smells like Indian food....Smells *Good*!" and my husband wanted to take some to work for his lunch. Pretty awesome.

On the second day of the cleanse, my husband wanted some of the food I made. Pretty cool. He ate it all and said, "Yeah, it's good." Who hoo!

My health is important, but getting my husband and the kids on board to better health is as well!

CHAPTER 5

Getting Your Family and Friends
on The Plan

Inspire Everyone to Be Healthier

Denise, 47

My six- and nine-year-old boys helped pack their lunches today. At least half of the items *they* chose were on The Plan. I love how eating healthy is not just helping me feel better, but is affecting my family in positive ways as well. Hubby is drinking more water and knocking out a few exercises as well. The boys will exercise with him at home, too. Since we only need to do twenty minutes or so, we can do it together as a family!

The Plan is eating what you love and what works for your chemistry. I want the whole family to eat according to this method because it helps in every aspect imaginable. In the beginning it may be hard to explain to them, but I know you can find a way to do it.

So does the whole family *really* get on board? In my experience and from what I've seen with our Plan clients and readers: Yes, they do! They may not want to jump in on Day One, but they can certainly join in on the Day Three dinner, when the food starts to feel more familiar to them. Of course your family may just surprise you! I hear from so many clients and readers that one of the things they love the most about The Plan is that they don't have to make separate meals for themselves and everyone else in their family. The recipes in this book are good for you, but they are also just plain good! With delicious meals, it won't be hard to bring the whole family around.

Lorraine, 46

I have included the whole family on The Plan dinners, making extra portions so that I could share it with them. The *big* upside is that everyone (and I mean everyone—including my picky four-year-old) is eating more veggies! I'm one super-happy mama—my son ate *kale,* zucchini, and broccoli! And I didn't have to make a ton of different meals to please everyone!

Here's what I want you to know. The more processed foods you allow your kids and family to eat, the more real food will taste foreign to them. But you can quickly change that! If meals until now have been mostly out of a box or the fast-food window, don't sweat it. Just start introducing The Plan meals to them and they will actually start *craving* healthier, less-processed foods. It's very important that everyone feels they have some ownership in this, and people are really more adventurous than we give them credit for.

I want everyone to enjoy the foods together and reap the health benefits! I have received thousands of emails from clients and readers saying how great The Plan has been for the family. Their kids have improved behavior, better attention spans, and better moods and hormonal balance. They see smaller waistlines, better blood work, and increased joyfulness in their mates. We get whole families on board, even friends and coworkers.

Louise, 52

My wife, Kim, and I love The Plan. We were dragged in kicking and screaming by my sister and her husband. And now I'm such an advocate, my boss and our in-house counsel are both doing The Plan with their partners and I talk about it to everyone. My sister's migraines are gone, my boss's wife's digestive problems are basically gone, my reflux is basically gone, and my blood pressure, cholesterol, and blood sugar are all down. Doctors are happy and so am I!

Sometimes you need to start a little slower and ease your family into The Plan, so let's not think about what they won't eat, but what they do like! Pasta and meatballs? Great, start with Mama's Mini Lamb Meatballs (page 179) and Low-Reactive Tomato Sauce (page 137), then add regular pasta and cut ribbons of baby romaine for a garnish. In two months, that pasta can be zucchini pasta (see page 100) and that garnish can be basil or sautéed kale ribbons.

Instead of sodium- and preservative-rich chicken fingers, dig into Panko-Crusted Chicken Tenders (page 170). Love cheesy, tomatoey goodness? Make Healthy Chicken Parmesan (page 167). Switch beef burgers to Lamb Burgers (page 177)—this is a popular one for families on The Plan. Chinese takeout turns into Spicy Orange Beef (page 182) or a simple Chicken Pad Thai with Zucchini Pasta (page 166) which you slowly add new veggies to. Katie's Kale Chips (page 119) are great, and so many more veggies might be more loved with our healthy Dairy-Free Ranch Dressing (page 150)!

Serving meals family style is a great way to allow everyone to find the foods they want and cut down on your time making separate dinners for everyone. Think of your table as one big salad bar, and you can use the leftovers for lunch the next day. One kid loves steamed broccoli and carrots, and the other likes a big salad with avocado and Plan Pizza (page 161)? Make one big quick-to-make smorgasbord and let them dig in. In fact, allowing kids to make more choices and having them be part of the process allows them to "own" their foods. I always see even the pickiest eater start to branch out when they have ownership in this way.

Jamie, 49

Just as you said, Lyn-Genet, my hot flashes have abated!! I am so happy and am now sleeping through the night every night. My cholesterol has dropped 62 points and my partner is amazed at how happy I am. To top it all off my synthroid has been reduced in half. In six weeks! I am so happy to not feel like I am battling my body and I now understand how to eat for me!

My mom and dad went on TP first and then my partner and I started after having dinner with them and seeing how much weight they lost! The ripple effect is amazing, because now my kids are on board. My youngest son is loving helping me cook and bake, my kids are making healthier choices for lunches and snacks, and we decided to start our own herb and vegetable garden this year! I can't believe it, but it feels like we have grown closer through this process.

Cutting Costs

In the first few weeks of Planning or making Plan meals you may wind up having to stock a whole pantry with new foods, and that's an investment up front. But I have heard time and time again that people have reduced their food costs overall by eating Plan friendly. In fact, many Planners have said that this new way of eating not only lessens their footprint on the planet, but has reduced their food cost as much as 30 percent! Of course there's the bonus of reduced medication and supplement costs as well!

Many of the foods on The Plan can be found at stores with discounted prices like Costco, Walmart, and Trader Joe's, and so many other grocery markets are now selling foods in bulk. I was shocked to see all of my "hard to find hippie foods" like hemp seeds and almond flour in a local grocery store in Texas at incredibly reasonable prices! Amazon.com has competitive prices and will ship anywhere, making your mailbox a cutting-edge grocery store no matter where you live.

If everyone in the family is eating the same food there is less waste, and that is invaluable on many levels. Buying in bulk is a great way to lower costs, especially when food is on sale. I find that purchasing the FoodSaver vacuum sealer has saved me thousands of dollars and freed up many hours of the daily task of cooking. It's so handy for making big portions of your favorite meals to freeze on the days that you *do* have time to cook. Busy week coming up? Break out those frozen meals you have made. You'll be eating healthier and saving money on takeout. I also love that their bags are BPA free!

I had lots of guests over for the Super Bowl at my house so I made the usual stuff and Plan-friendly food. My mother-in-law loved the Vegetable Timbale; she even asked for the recipe! She also loved the kale chips—she had never had kale before! She was amazed that the kids ate more kale chips and carrots instead of the potato chips and tortilla chips. She also had lamb for the first time last night when I made the Mama's Mini Lamb Meatballs. I think she is going to make my father-in-law make the Vegetable Timbale as soon as they get home!

Sample Plan-Friendly Menus

Worried about pleasing friends and family during holidays and other celebrations while following The Plan? No need! Here are some easy crowd-pleasing menus you can put together with the recipes in this book. Enjoy!

Thanksgiving Dinner Menu
Thanksgiving Mini Muffins (page 189)
Warm Dandelion Salad (page 100)
Roasted Vegetable, Frisee, and Manchego Salad (page 97)
Roast Chicken (page 171) with Persian Pomegranate Sauce (page 140)
Lamb Shepherd's Pie (page 176)
Apple Streusel (page 197)

Christmas Dinner Menu
Goat Cheese Trio (page 117)
Shiitake Pâté (page 118)
Prime Rib (page 183)
Cornish Game Hens (page 172)
Panko-Crusted Brussels Sprouts (page 124)
Radicchio and Pomegranate Salad (page 96)
So Rich You Could Die Chocolate Pie (page 193)

July 4th Menu
Grilled Vegetable Salad (page 92)
Mediterranean Grilled Lamb Chops (page 179)
Calamari Salad (page 90)
Kale, Avocado, and Cranberry Salad (page 94)
Watermelon Caprese (page 93)

Super Bowl Menu
Jalapeño Poppers (page 127)
Grilled Turmeric Chicken Wings (page 129)
Dairy-Free Ranch Dressing (page 150) with crudités

5-Layer Dip (page 114)

Vegetable Timbale (page 125)

Katie's Kale Chips (page 119)

Summer Brunch Menu

Huevos Rancheros (page 81)

Gluten-Free Blueberry Muffins (page 80)

Avocado Fries with Sweet 'n' Sour Sauce (page 121)

Butternut Squash Pancakes (page 72)

Breakfast

Do you really need to eat breakfast? Depends. I'm sure by now you must have figured out that I don't always have black-and-white answers! It depends on what works for *you*. Some of my clients wake up hungry. They should eat. Some of my clients aren't hungry until 10 a.m. and that's when they should eat. It's really that simple.

Eating later should mean structuring your day a little differently. Maybe you should have lunch later. Have a snack if you're hungry, don't if you're not. We have really lost the art of listening to the brain in our stomach and have let the brain in our cranium take over. That's not the wisest choice when it comes to food. Start listening to your gut and you will find you will make the best choices.

Writing this reminds me of when there was the first batch of articles coming out about The Plan and I said, "Oatmeal is the devil!" My inbox was *inundated* with people saying, "Thank God you said that. I'd eat oatmeal, feel bloated, sluggish, and blah all day, but I kept eating it because I was told it's the healthy thing to do. I *hate* oatmeal. Now I can give it up."

We have come to a sad place if we are forcing ourselves to ignore our body's innate intelligence because we are told by "experts" that we *have* to eat something. Remember your body is always talking to you. Start listening and your weight and health will fall into line.

Here's a good way to gauge if your breakfast is working for you: You're pleasantly full for 3 to 4 hours after you eat: not too stuffed and certainly not able to go the whole day without eating! (When that happens you ate a food that was too tough for your body to digest. If something is reactive, your body may shut down hunger so it can take extra time to break down the problematic food.)

And what if the opposite happens? When you are *starving* after breakfast? That usually means there wasn't enough protein or fat or there was too much sugar in your breakfast. You are unique and your protein needs at breakfast will vary depending on your chemistry. Ghrelin, the hunger hormone, is kept in check when you eat enough protein. Here are some ranges of protein to have at breakfast for women and men:

Women: 10 to 40 grams of protein
Men: 15 to 60 grams of protein

Low-Reactive Vegetarian Sources of Protein
Sunflower seeds: 5 grams per ounce (these are also good sources of calcium!)
Pumpkin seeds: 9 grams per ounce (great source of zinc for your immune system!)

Almonds: 8 grams per ounce

Basmati or brown rice: 6 grams per cup

Chia seeds: 5 grams per 2 tablespoons (a great source of omega-3s!)

Hemp seeds: 11 grams per 3 tablespoons (great for iron, magnesium, potassium, and zinc)

Spelt: 1 cup cooked = 11 grams

Flax seeds: 16 grams per half cup (and 23 grams of fiber!)

Now before you start worrying about calculating fat, the good news is that when you meet the protein requirements you have likely eaten just enough fat, too. Some other helpful tips: Stay within the protein ranges unless you are very athletic, don't overthink it, and listen to your gut!

Eggs are higher on the reactive scale (almost 40 percent of Planners react to eggs), so definitely note how you feel on them if you haven't done the full twenty-day Plan. This section has plenty of other options for breakfast that will provide you with clean-burning fuel for your day!

Kamut and spelt are very similar to wheat but easier to digest for most folks, so definitely keep that in mind if you think wheat may be a slight problem for you. Arrowhead Mills makes great low-sodium, low-sugar cereals that are a perfect breakfast if you add some sunflower seeds or almonds to them. Kamut and spelt flakes are getting easier to find as people become aware of their food sensitivities. Rice flakes are also a super-friendly breakfast option. We do find that many popped or puffed cereals can be a problem as they are processed at a high heat, so keep an eye on that!

As for flax, flax granola can be funny. There are the people who *hate* it and suffer through it for five days; and then two weeks later they don't want to eat anything else. Then there's the group that love it from Day One and become addicts. I am telling both of you, please limit flax to twice a week after the first couple of weeks of The Plan. Flax is a phytoestrogen and in small amounts really does help our bodies balance out hormones. But as soon as you start to consume it too often it can start to skew our hormonal balance, for men and women!

What my team and I have really found out is that rotating your foods is the most important thing you can do for your health. Every food, and I mean every food, has its health benefits and potential health risks. If you keep changing the stimulus with your friendly foods your body will get the variety of nutrients it needs and this will help your body to nourish and heal.

PLAN SMOOTHIE

To ripen pears quickly, place them on a windowsill in sunlight; they will be ripe the next day. Organic pears are often much less expensive than organic apples. Frozen mango and frozen blueberries can be a great time-saver and they are often less expensive than fresh.

    1 cup Silk coconut milk or Rice Dream
    1 cup blueberries
    ½ cup chopped pear or mango
    ¼ avocado
    ¼ cup chia seeds
    Optional: 1 tsp honey or agave nectar
    Optional: ½ tsp pure vanilla extract
    Optional: ½ tsp ground cinnamon, or to taste

Combine all ingredients in a blender and blend until smooth (you can add ice, too, but it is not recommended if you have thyroid dysfunction).

Makes 1 serving

FLAX GRANOLA

A plan staple, chock-full of protein, omega-3s, calcium, and fiber.

    1 cup water
    2 cups whole flaxseeds
    1 tbsp agave nectar
    2 tsp ground cinnamon
    1 tsp ground cardamom

1 tsp pure vanilla extract

½ tsp nutmeg

½ cup raisins

Combine water and flaxseeds in a medium bowl and mix well. Let sit for 30 minutes and mix again.

Preheat oven to 275°F. Add agave, cinnamon, cardamom, vanilla, and nutmeg to flaxseeds and mix thoroughly.

Spread granola in a thin layer on a baking sheet and bake for 50 minutes. Reduce oven temperature to 225°F. Cut sheet of granola into clusters, flip, and bake an additional 30 to 40 minutes, until thoroughly dry. Add raisins and store in airtight container. Consume within 2 weeks.

Makes 2 to 4 servings (about 4 cups)

WARM SPELT FLAKES WITH MANGO-BLUEBERRY COMPOTE

Spelt is similar to wheat but easier for many people to digest. Bob's Red Mill makes great spelt flakes. You can also find spelt flakes in bulk sections of health food stores for even greater savings.

4 cups spelt flakes

3¼ cups water

1 cup chopped mango (fresh or frozen)

½ cup blueberries (fresh or frozen)

1 tbsp honey or agave nectar

1 tsp fresh lemon juice

½ tsp grated peeled fresh ginger

Soak spelt flakes in 3 cups water in a large bowl in the refrigerator overnight. (Soaking makes the spelt flakes even more digestible.)

The next day, in a small saucepan, combine mango, blueberries, honey or agave, lemon juice, ginger, and ¼ cup more water. Bring to a boil over high heat. Lower the heat and simmer until the fruit is softened and the liquid thickened, about 15 minutes. Serve warm spelt cereal with mango-blueberry sauce.

Yields 4 servings

WARM RAISIN FLAX CEREAL

Perfect for a cold winter morning, this hot cereal will warm your bones.

1 cup whole flaxseeds
1 cup water
¼ cup raisins
½ cup Rice Dream
1 tbsp honey
1 tsp ground cinnamon
½ tsp cardamom
¼ tsp nutmeg

Soak flaxseeds in the water overnight in a bowl.

The next day, combine the soaked flaxseeds, raisins, Rice Dream, honey, cinnamon, cardamom, and nutmeg in a saucepan over low heat. Simmer for 1 to 2 minutes, until thoroughly warmed. Enjoy immediately.

Makes 2 to 3 servings

APPLE PANCAKES

1 cup whole wheat flour
1 tsp baking powder
⅛ tsp baking soda
1 tsp ground cinnamon
½ tsp nutmeg

Dash of ground cloves

2 tbsp chia seeds

1 cup Silk vanilla coconut milk or Vanilla Rice Dream (see Note)

1 tbsp unsalted butter, softened, plus more for greasing

1 large egg

1 tsp pure vanilla extract

1 cup grated apple

In a medium bowl, whisk together flour, baking powder, baking soda, cinnamon, nutmeg, cloves, and chia seeds. In a large glass measuring cup or small bowl, whisk together coconut milk or Rice Dream, 1 tbsp softened butter, egg, and vanilla. Pour wet ingredients over dry ingredients and whisk until combined. Add apple and whisk until combined.

Heat a pan or griddle over medium-low heat; melt a little butter; ladle batter into pan ¼ cup at a time, spacing the pancakes a few inches from each other. When pancakes start to bubble (after 2 minutes), flip and cook another 2 minutes, until pancakes are lightly browned on both sides. Repeat with the remaining batter.

Note: You can use plain Silk coconut milk or Rice Dream; just add 1 to 2 tbsp brown sugar to the batter to make the pancakes sweeter.

Makes 3 to 4 servings (6 to 8 pancakes)

BERRY PROTEIN CAKES

¼ cup (½ stick) unsalted butter, softened, plus more for greasing

2 cups all-purpose flour

2 tsp baking powder

½ tsp baking soda

1 tsp ground cinnamon

½ tsp allspice

2 large eggs

½ cup honey

½ cup Silk coconut milk or Rice Dream

4 cups blueberries

¼ cup whole flaxseeds

2 tbsp chia seeds

2 tbsp sunflower seeds

Preheat oven to 375°F. Butter a 12-cup muffin tin.

Combine flour, baking powder, baking soda, cinnamon, and allspice in a medium mixing bowl. In a separate bowl, whisk together eggs, honey, coconut milk or Rice Dream, and ¼ cup butter. Pour wet ingredients into dry and mix well. Stir in berries and seeds.

Pour batter into cups of prepared muffin tin and bake for about 15 minutes, until an inserted toothpick comes out clean.

Makes 12 servings

BUTTERNUT SQUASH PANCAKES

The flour and butternut squash will give you a lot of fuel on days you work out. It's a great breakfast for runners!

2 cups all-purpose flour

1 tsp baking powder

½ tsp baking soda

1 tsp ground cinnamon

½ tsp cardamom

⅛ tsp nutmeg

2 tbsp chia seeds

Optional: 2 tbsp almond slivers

¾ cup pureed cooked butternut squash

1¼ cups Silk coconut milk or Rice Dream (see Note)

1 tbsp unsalted butter, softened, plus more for greasing

2 large eggs

½ tsp pure vanilla extract

Combine flour, baking powder, baking soda, cinnamon, cardamom, nutmeg, and chia in a mixing bowl. Add almond slivers for extra protein, if desired. In a large bowl, whisk together squash, coconut milk or Rice Dream, 1 tbsp softened butter, eggs, and vanilla. Add dry mixture to wet and combine into a thick batter.

Heat a pan or griddle over medium-low heat; melt a little butter; ladle batter into pan, ¼ cup at a time. When pancakes start to bubble (after 2 minutes), flip and cook another 2 minutes until pancakes are lightly browned on both sides. Repeat with the remaining batter.

Note: You can use plain Silk coconut milk or Rice Dream; just add 1 to 2 tbsp brown sugar to the batter to make the pancakes sweeter.

Makes 6 to 8 servings (about 12 pancakes)

ZUCCHINI PANCAKES (*KOOKOO KADOO*)

I totally prefer saying this name in Turkish; it always brings a smile to kids' faces.

    4 cups shredded zucchini (from about 2 large zucchini)
    5 large eggs
    1 small onion, chopped
    2 to 3 cloves garlic, finely chopped
    ¼ cup coconut flour
    ¼ cup chopped fresh dill
    2 tbsp extra virgin olive oil
    Optional topping: ½ cup grated goat-cheese Gouda

Blot zucchini dry or squeeze in a towel to remove moisture. In a large mixing bowl, combine zucchini, eggs, onion, garlic, coconut flour, dill, and 1 tbsp olive oil and mix thoroughly.

Heat remaining 1 tbsp oil in a skillet over medium heat. Using half the batter, roughly form 8 pancakes in the skillet and cook until browned. Flip and cook on other side until browned, 2 to 3 minutes. Repeat with the remaining zucchini mix and add more oil if needed. Serve hot, with cheese if you like.

Makes 4 servings (16 small pancakes)

QUICK AND EASY BLUEBERRY COMPOTE

I don't know about you, but I don't have much time to prep. And sit. And let things gestate. So here's a quicker and updated version of my much beloved Blueberry Pear Compote.

    2 cups blueberries
    2¼ cups Silk coconut milk or Rice Dream
    1 cup chia seeds
    1 tbsp agave nectar
    1 tsp pure vanilla extract

½ tsp cardamom

½ cup almond slivers or sunflower seeds

Combine blueberries, coconut milk or Rice Dream, chia, agave, vanilla, and cardamom in a small saucepan and bring to a boil. Reduce heat to simmer and let simmer for 2 to 3 minutes, stirring constantly to prevent the chia from congealing. Let sit for 5 minutes for soft compote, 10 minutes for firmer compote.

Top with almond slivers or sunflower seeds. Serve warm.

Makes 4 servings (4 to 5 cups)

BUTTERNUT SQUASH SOUFFLÉ

This is another egg-rich dish, chock-full of protein, and your body can utilize these sugars for an a.m. workout!

3 tbsp unsalted butter, softened, plus more for greasing

2½ cups pureed cooked butternut squash

⅓ cup Silk coconut milk or Rice Dream

¼ cup packed brown sugar

1 tsp ground cinnamon

1 tsp nutmeg

½ tsp cardamom

⅛ tsp sea salt

3 large eggs

1 tsp pure vanilla extract

Preheat oven to 350°F. Lightly butter a 9x9-inch casserole dish.

In a food processor, combine butternut squash and 3 tbsp softened butter and puree until smooth. Add coconut milk or Rice Dream, brown sugar, cinnamon, nutmeg, cardamom, and salt and puree again. Add eggs and vanilla and puree for an additional minute.

Pour into prepared casserole dish. Bake for 25 to 30 minutes, until the crust is brown and the center jiggles just slightly when you shake it. Serve immediately.

Makes 4 servings

CHOCOLATE-CHIA POWER BREAKFAST CAKE

A great breakfast to make ahead for those days you barely have time to sit down. It's also delicious with nut butter.

1½ cups all-purpose flour

⅓ cup cocoa powder

2 tsp ground cinnamon

½ tsp nutmeg

¼ cup almond slivers

1¼ cups Vanilla Rice Dream

½ cup honey

½ cup (1 stick) unsalted butter, softened

¼ cup chia seeds

1 tsp pure vanilla extract

Preheat oven to 350°F.

Sift together flour, cocoa, cinnamon, and nutmeg into a medium bowl and add almonds. Add Rice Dream, honey, butter, chia, and vanilla to dry ingredients and stir well. Pour batter into an 8-inch-square baking pan. Bake for 35 minutes. Store in an airtight container and consume within 3 to 4 days.

Makes 8 to 10 servings

GINGER PEAR CRUMBLE

I prefer my desserts naturally sweetened; if you do too, try cutting down what is already a low-sugar breakfast by omitting the sugar.

Butter, for greasing the pie dish

Pear Filling

2 lb pears, cored and chopped into 1-inch pieces (from about 4 large pears)

1 cup fresh cranberries

3 tbsp brown sugar

3 tbsp chopped peeled fresh ginger (from 3-inch piece)

½ tsp grated organic lemon zest

Juice of ½ lemon (about 1½ tbsp)

½ tsp nutmeg

Crumble Topping

1 cup blanched almond flour

3 tbsp unsalted butter, softened

1 tbsp brown sugar

½ tsp ground cinnamon

½ tsp allspice

Preheat oven to 375°F. Butter a 9-inch pie dish.

To make pear filling, combine all ingredients in a large mixing bowl; transfer to prepared pie tin.

To make crumble, combine all ingredients in a small mixing bowl and stir well. Spread crumble on top of pear filling. Bake for 30 minutes, until crumble is browned. Let cool.

Makes 8 servings

CHIA HEMP PUDDING

This is a quick, protein-rich breakfast for vegans. Many Planners find they lose weight more quickly when they add hemp seeds to their meals.

½ cup chia seeds

2 cups water

1 cup shelled hemp seeds

2 tsp pure vanilla extract

2 tbsp agave nectar or honey

Dash of sea salt

Place chia seeds in a medium mixing bowl. Combine remaining ingredients in a blender or food processor and blend well. Let mixture sit in blender for 1 minute, then blend again for 30 seconds.

Pour contents over the chia in the mixing bowl. Let sit for 5 to 10 minutes. The chia seeds will start to release their magical mucilage and make the pudding firm. Serve at room temperature.

Makes 4 servings

PUMPKIN PIE–CHIA PUDDING

1 cup Silk coconut milk or Rice Dream

1 cup canned or pureed cooked pumpkin, chilled if possible

½ cup chia seeds

1 tbsp maple syrup

½ tsp ground cinnamon, or more to taste

¼ tsp ground ginger

Pinch of nutmeg

Dash of pure vanilla extract

Place all ingredients in a food processor or blender and blend to combine. Let pudding sit for 5 to 10 minutes at room temperature for soft pudding, or 20 minutes for firmer pudding.

Makes 2 to 4 servings

RICE PUDDING (*KHEER*)

This warming breakfast is great to fuel your day or your morning run. Serve with nuts or seeds of your choice to boost protein.

2 cups cooked basmati rice

1 cup Silk coconut milk or Rice Dream

¼ cup raisins

1 tsp cinnamon

½ tsp cardamom

½ tsp ground ginger

Optional: ½ tsp rose water

In a medium saucepan, combine all ingredients over low heat and simmer, stirring frequently, 3 to 4 minutes, until well mixed and fragrant. Serve warm.

Makes 4 to 6 servings

ZUCCHINI BREAD

¼ cup (½ stick) unsalted butter, softened, plus more for greasing

¼ cup honey

1 large egg

¼ cup unsweetened applesauce

2 cups shredded zucchini (from about 1 large zucchini)

2 tsp grated organic lemon zest

2 tbsp lemon juice

1½ cups all-purpose flour

½ tsp baking soda

¼ tsp baking powder

1 tsp ground cinnamon

Preheat oven to 325°F. Grease an 8x4-inch loaf pan.

In a bowl, beat together honey, egg, applesauce, and ¼ cup softened butter. Blot zucchini dry or squeeze in towel to remove excess water. Stir zucchini, lemon zest, and lemon juice into honey mixture.

In a separate bowl, sift together flour, baking soda, baking powder, and cinnamon. Stir flour mixture into zucchini mixture just until blended.

Pour batter into prepared pan. Bake for 45 minutes, until a knife inserted in the center comes out clean. Cool about 10 minutes before turning out onto a wire rack to cool completely.

Makes 8 to 10 servings

GLUTEN-FREE RAISIN CINNAMON BREAD

While you can use leftover ground almonds for an almond flour, using blanched flour gives such a lighter texture!

    ¼ cup (½ stick) unsalted butter, softened, plus more for greasing

    2 cups blanched almond flour

    ½ tsp baking soda

    2 tbsp ground cinnamon

    ½ tsp cardamom

    Pinch of ground cloves

    5 large eggs

    ¼ cup raisins

    2 tbsp honey

    2 tbsp applesauce

    1 tsp pure vanilla extract

Preheat oven to 350°F. Butter an 8x4-inch loaf pan.

In a medium bowl, combine almond flour, baking soda, cinnamon, cardamom, and cloves and mix thoroughly. In a large bowl, combine eggs, ¼ cup softened butter, raisins, honey, applesauce, and vanilla and mix thoroughly. Slowly add dry ingredients to wet. Mix thoroughly.

Pour batter into prepared loaf pan. Bake for 30 to 35 minutes, until a toothpick inserted into the center comes out clean. Let cool slightly and serve warm.

Makes 8 servings

GLUTEN-FREE BLUEBERRY MUFFINS

These muffins are egg rich, so make sure that eggs are friendly for you before you try them.

    ½ cup (1 stick) unsalted butter, softened, plus more for greasing

    ½ cup coconut flour

½ tsp baking soda

Dash of sea salt

6 large eggs

½ cup honey

1 tbsp pure vanilla extract

1 cup blueberries (fresh or frozen)

Preheat oven to 350°F. Generously butter a 6-cup muffin tin.

In a small bowl, combine coconut flour, baking soda, and salt. In a large bowl, whisk eggs, honey, ½ cup softened butter, and vanilla. Mix dry ingredients into wet. Gently fold in blueberries.

Spoon batter into cups of prepared muffin tin. Bake for 20 to 25 minutes, until inserted toothpick comes out clean. Cool and serve.

Makes 6 servings

HUEVOS RANCHEROS

Eating brunch out can be such a weight gain experience! Turn that around by inviting friends over. Serve this hearty dish paired with seasonal fruit and a basket of cinnamon raisin bread, gluten-free muffins, and your beverage of choice.

6 large eggs

2 tbsp extra virgin olive oil

12 Veg Chia Crisps (page 120)

½ cup Quick and Easy Ranchero Sauce (page 148)

Optional toppings: ¾ cup Plan Guacamole (page 114), ¾ cup chopped lettuce, ½ cup grated goat-cheese Cheddar

Whisk eggs in a mixing bowl for 30 seconds. Heat a skillet over medium heat and add oil. Pour eggs into skillet and scramble to desired consistency.

Place 3 chia crackers on each of 4 plates and top with scrambled eggs, ranchero sauce, and any desired toppings.

Makes 4 servings

ALMOND GRABBERS

These make a great breakfast when you are on the run or just need a nice protein-rich snack.

1 cup almond slivers

½ cup coconut flakes

¼ cup raw almond butter

2 tbsp honey

2 tbsp chia seeds

2 tbsp whole flaxseeds

2 tbsp rice milk

1 tsp pure vanilla extract

Preheat oven to 375°F.

In a medium bowl, combine all ingredients together. Let mixture sit for 15 minutes for the chia to release mucilage. If the dough isn't sticky enough, add a dash more rice milk.

Form mixture into 2-inch balls and place on an ungreased baking sheet. Bake for 15 minutes, but check at 12 minutes: If tops are golden brown, they are done. Let cool. Store in an airtight container and consume within one week

Makes 10 servings (20 balls)

RICE MILK HORCHATA

5 cups water

1¼ cups uncooked basmati rice

1 tsp pure vanilla extract

½ tsp ground cinnamon

Optional: 2 tbsp brown sugar

Combine all ingredients in a medium saucepan and cook over low heat for 30 to 40 minutes, until the rice is a porridge-type texture. Let cool.

Transfer to blender or food processor and blend for 2 to 3 minutes. Let stand for 45 minutes.

Strain mixture through a cheesecloth into a widemouthed quart mason jar. (The solids may be thrown away or used for rice pudding.)

Makes 4 servings

ALMOND MILK

Almond milk from a carton is 60 percent reactive and filled with preservatives. Try this version and see how much better you feel!

2 cups raw almonds

5 cups water

Optional: 2 tbsp honey, sugar, agave nectar, or maple syrup

Optional: 2 tbsp pure vanilla extract

Special equipment: Fine-mesh nut bag or cheesecloth

Soak almonds overnight in 3 cups water.

Drain and rinse almonds. Combine 2 cups water and almonds in a food processor and blend at highest speed for 4 minutes, pausing occasionally to scrape bowl and combine all almonds for better processing. Pour almond mixture into a strainer lined with cheesecloth and placed over any receptacle (large enough to hold 5 cups). Strain almond milk until most of the liquid is in container. Squeeze out the rest of the almond milk by wringing cheesecloth.

Taste almond milk and add sweetener and/or vanilla, if desired. Refrigerate in sealed containers for up to 2 days.

Note: Leftover almond meal can be used as a coarse-grain almond flour when dried at low heat (225°F) for 2 to 3 hours.

Makes 4 servings (4 cups)

ALMOND BUTTER

The trick to making good almond butter is to roast your almonds first, which releases the oils. It is best to roast the almonds the day before or let them have time to cool.

3 cups raw almonds
4 to 5 tbsp extra virgin olive oil

Preheat oven to 250°F. Spread almonds on an ungreased baking sheet and bake for 30 minutes. Let cool for 30 minutes or up to 24 hours.

Process almonds in a food processor on high until they begin to form a ball. Drizzle olive oil over almonds and continue to blend, scraping sides of bowl with a spatula as needed. Store in an airtight container for up to 1 week.

Makes 10 to 16 servings (2 cups)

APPLE-CINNAMON ALMOND BUTTER

When it comes to feeding some kids, it's all about sneaking in the extra nutrients like apples and cinnamon when you can. Actually it's that way with a lot of adults, too! Unless you make your own almond butter, please remember that store-bought roasted almond butter is higher reactive, so note how you feel after eating it.

1 cup raw or homemade Almond Butter (above)
¼ cup applesauce
1 tsp ground cinnamon

Place all ingredients in a food processor and blend for 1 to 2 minutes, until fully combined. Transfer to an airtight container and refrigerate for up to 1 week. Great on pancakes or toast.

Makes 8 to 10 servings (about 1¼ cups)

SUNFLOWER BUTTER

Unfortunately I have never seen raw sunflower butter in a store, so you may want to try making your own to decrease potential for reactivity!

2 cups unsalted hulled raw sunflower seeds

2 tbsp extra virgin olive oil

Preheat oven to 250°F.

Spread sunflower seeds on a large baking sheet in a thin layer. Bake for 10 minutes. Stir seeds and bake for another 5 minutes, until lightly browned. Let cool for 30 minutes or up to 24 hours.

Transfer roasted seeds to a food processor or high-powered blender (such as a Vitamix). Blend or pulse for a total of 5 to 7 minutes, until thoroughly blended. Let rest for 5 minutes so oils can seep out from seeds. Restart blending slowly, adding in olive oil. Total blending time will be 12 to 15 minutes. Store in an airtight container in the fridge for up to 7 to 10 days.

Makes 20 servings (1¾ cups)

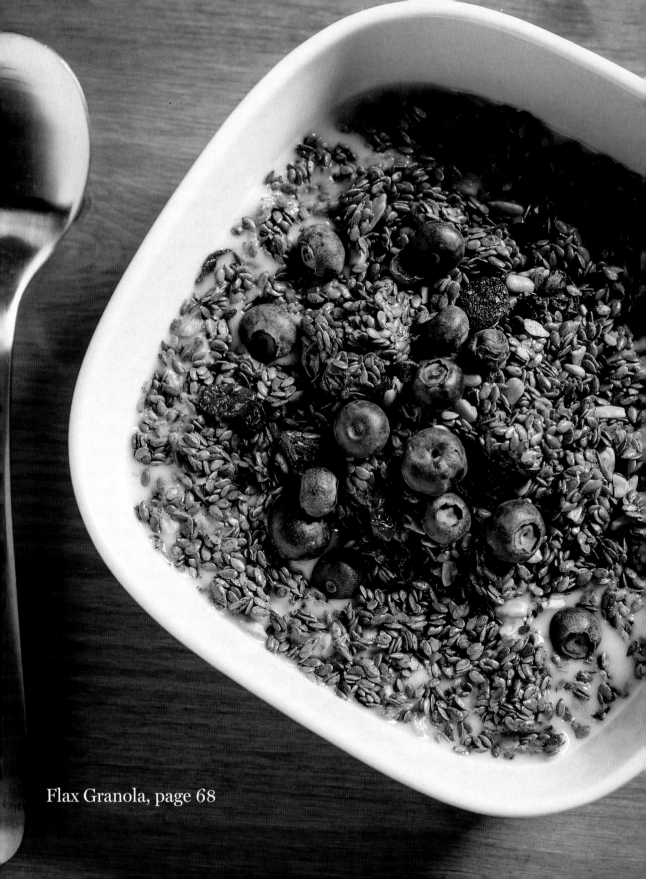

Flax Granola, page 68

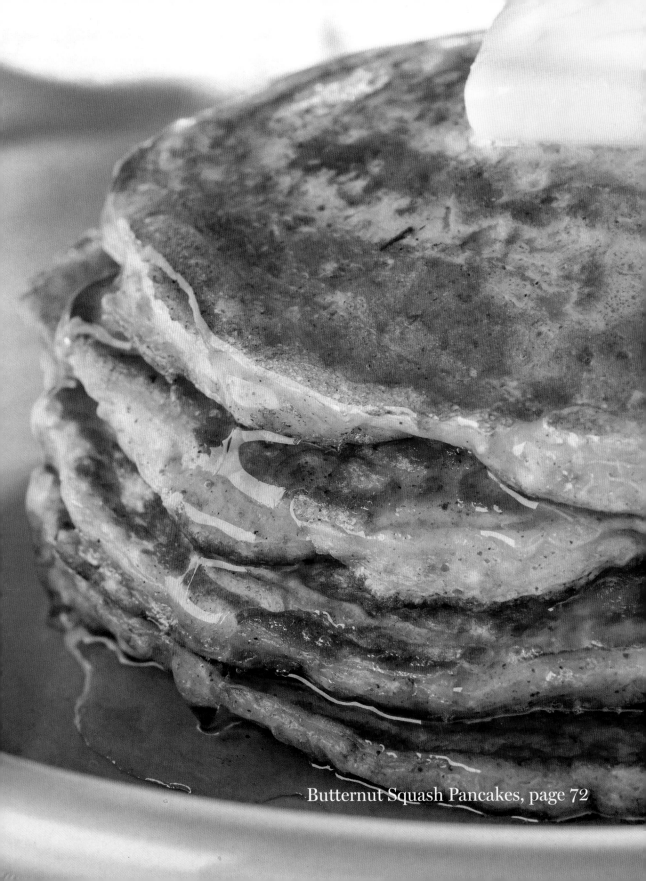

Butternut Squash Pancakes, page 72

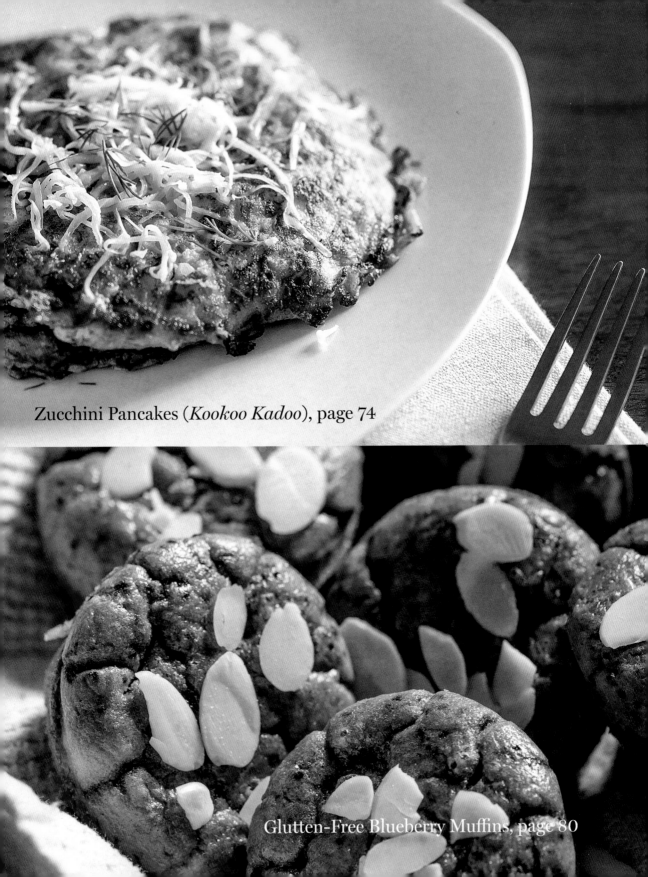

Zucchini Pancakes (*Kookoo Kadoo*), page 74

Glutten-Free Blueberry Muffins, page 80

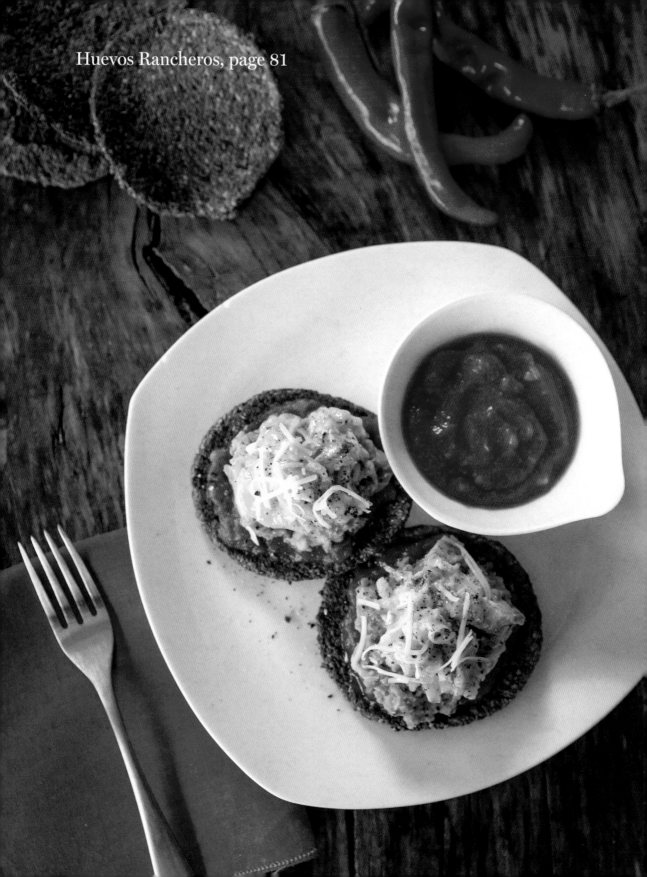

Huevos Rancheros, page 81

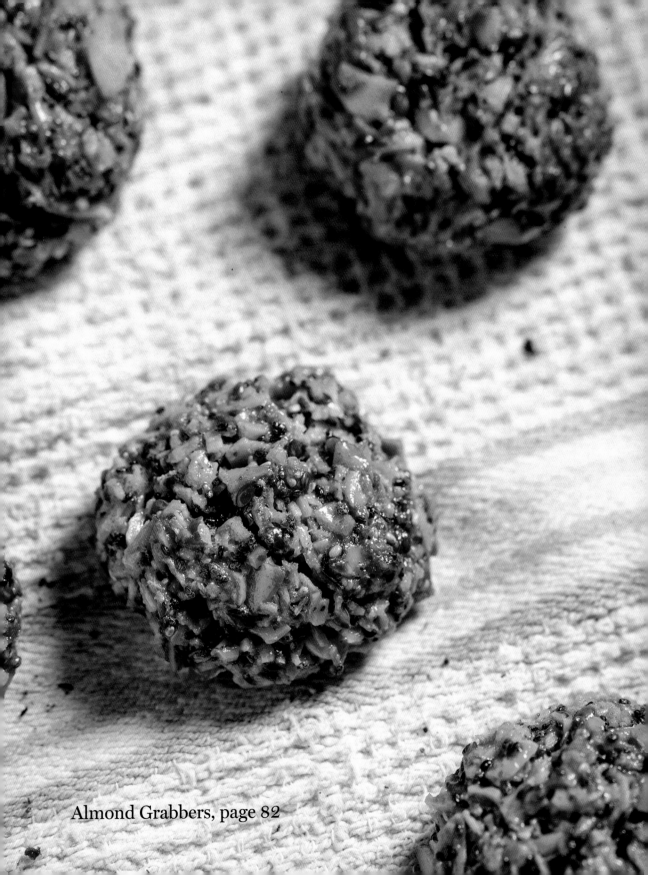

Almond Grabbers, page 82

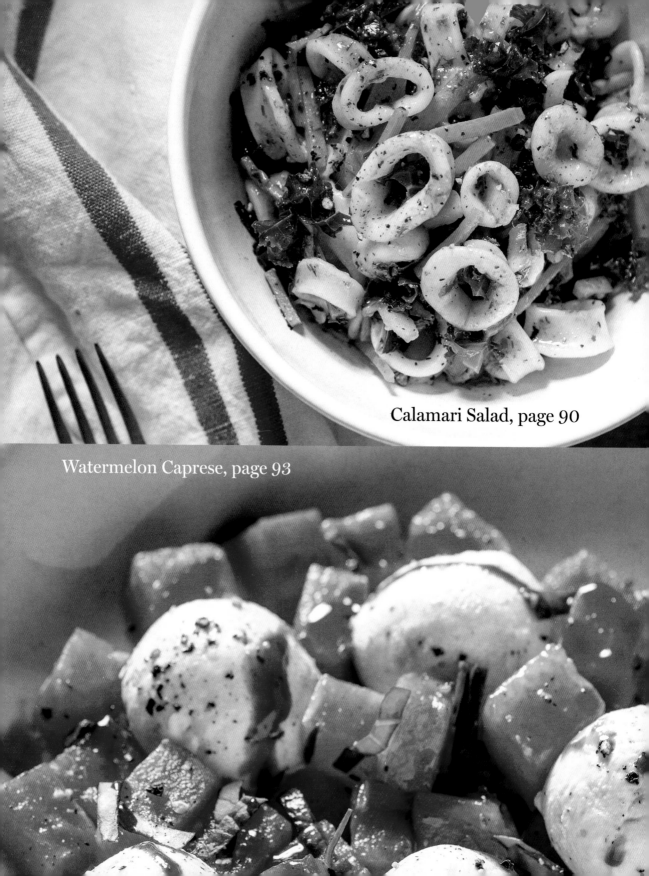

Calamari Salad, page 90

Watermelon Caprese, page 93

Israeli Salad, page 93, with Creamy Cucumber Sauce, page 139

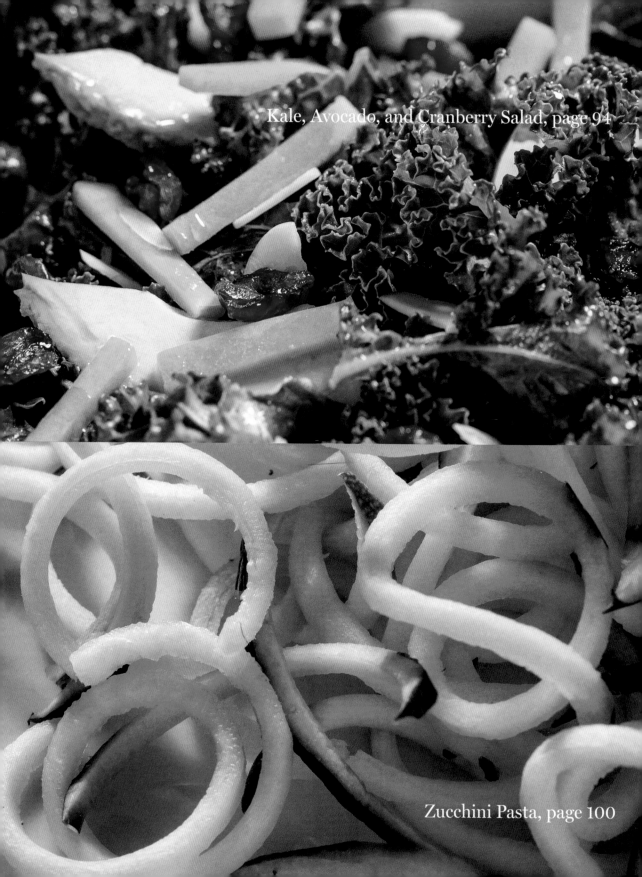

Kale, Avocado, and Cranberry Salad, page 94

Zucchini Pasta, page 100

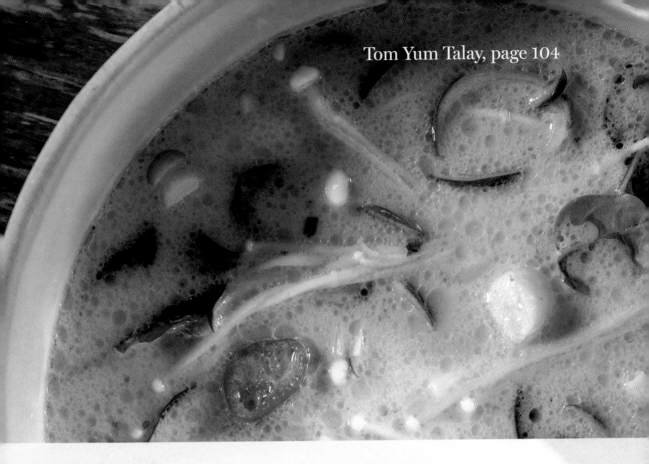
Tom Yum Talay, page 104

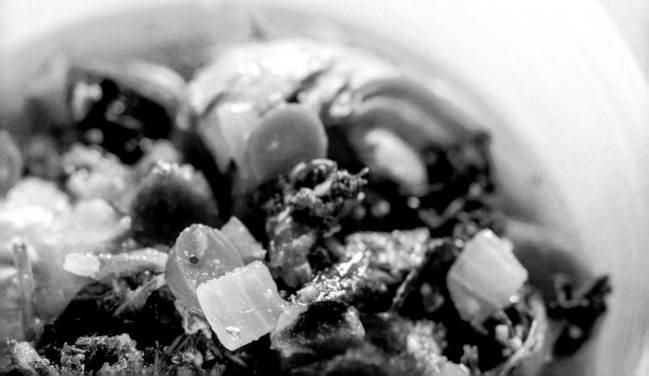
Slow Cooker Chicken "Noodle" Soup, page 106

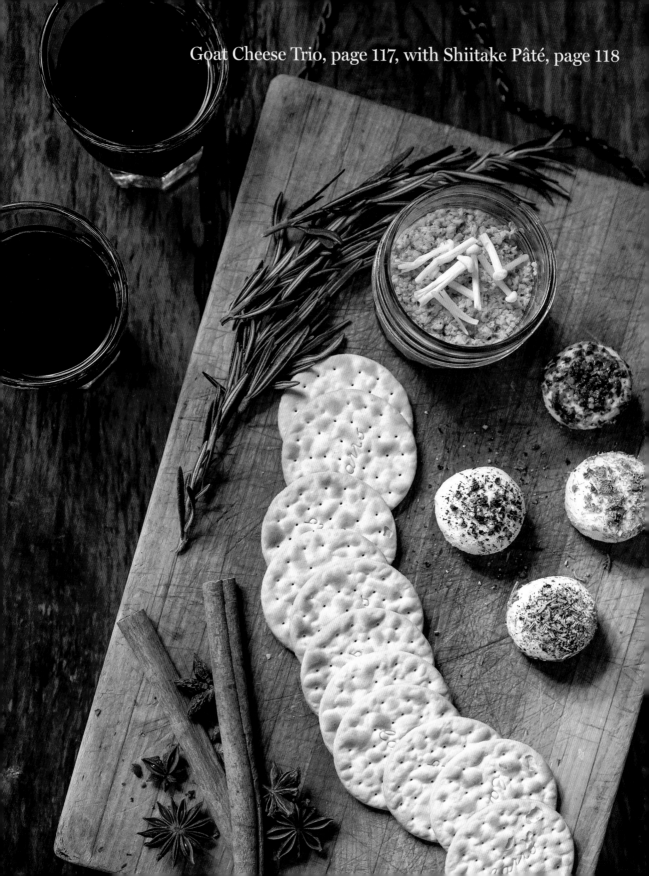

Goat Cheese Trio, page 117, with Shiitake Pâté, page 118

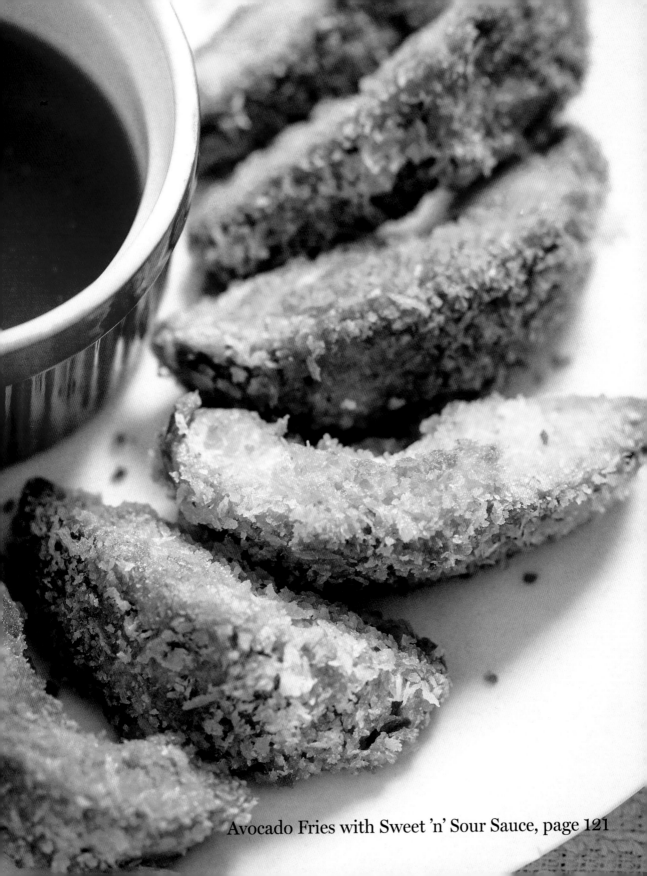

Avocado Fries with Sweet 'n' Sour Sauce, page 121

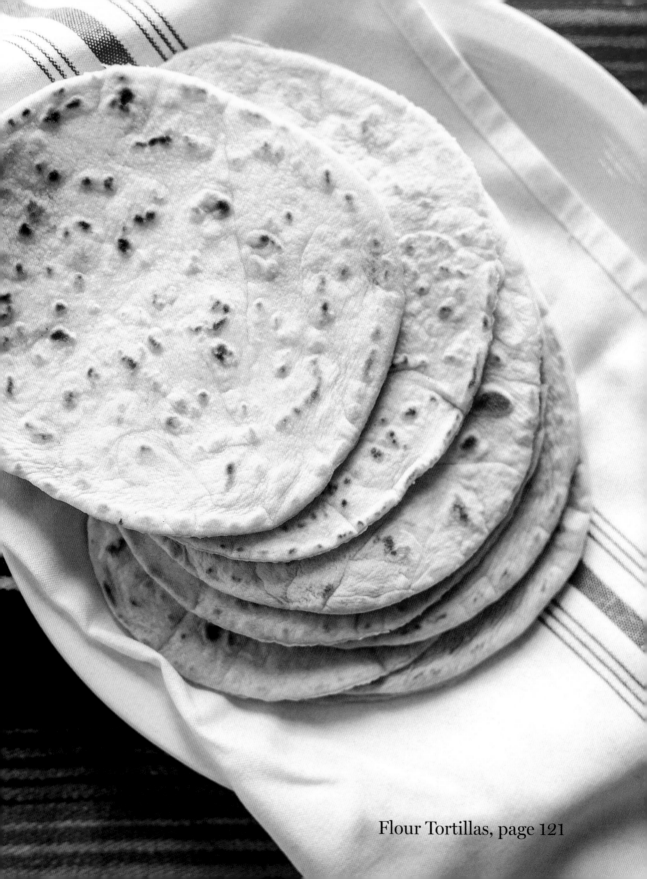

Flour Tortillas, page 121

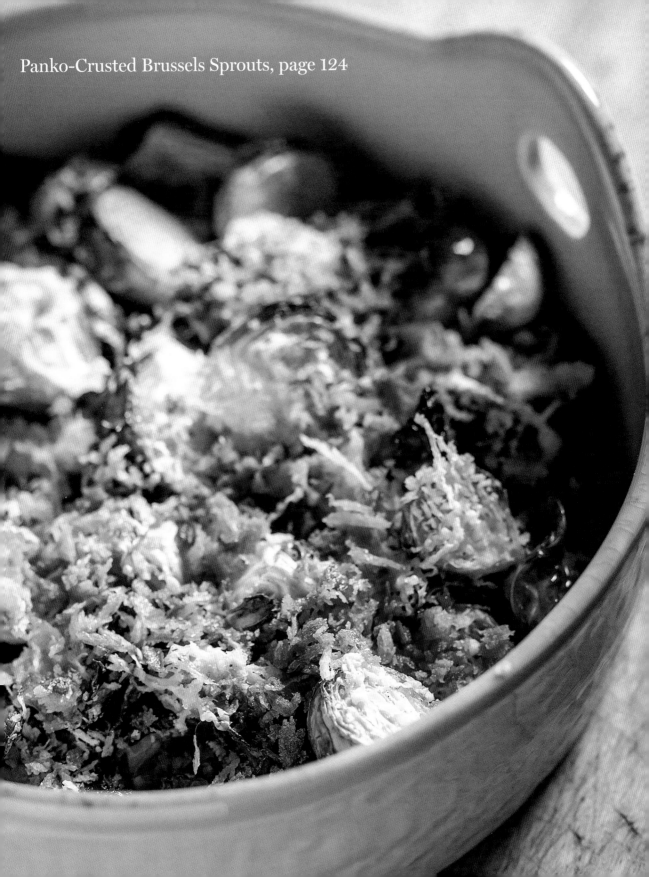

Panko-Crusted Brussels Sprouts, page 124

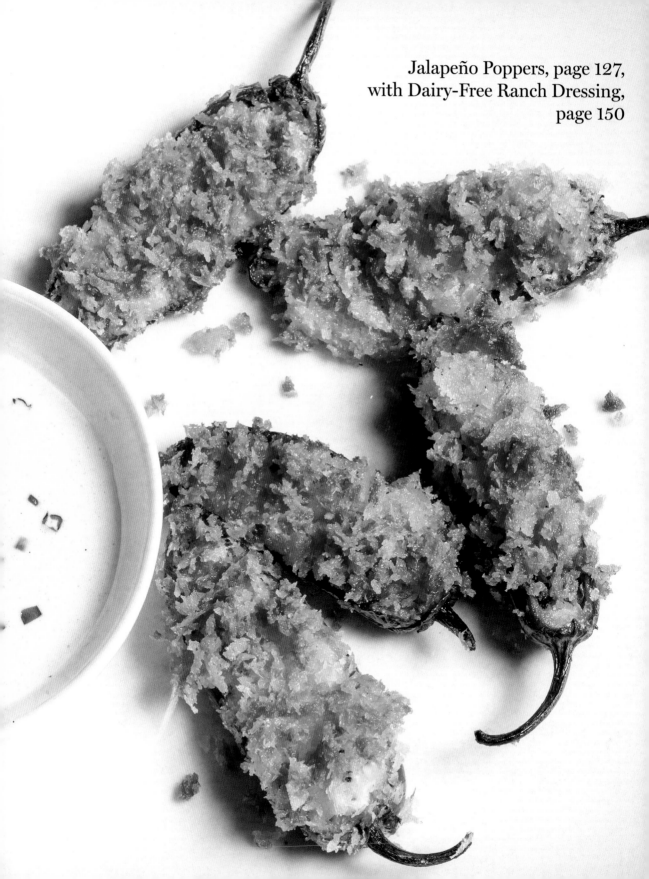

Jalapeño Poppers, page 127, with Dairy-Free Ranch Dressing, page 150

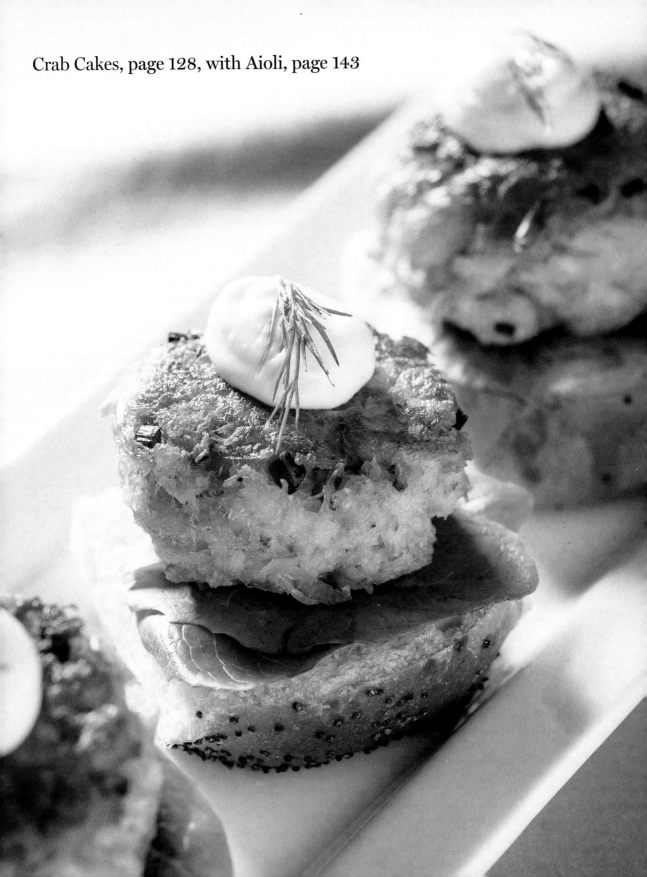

Crab Cakes, page 128, with Aioli, page 143

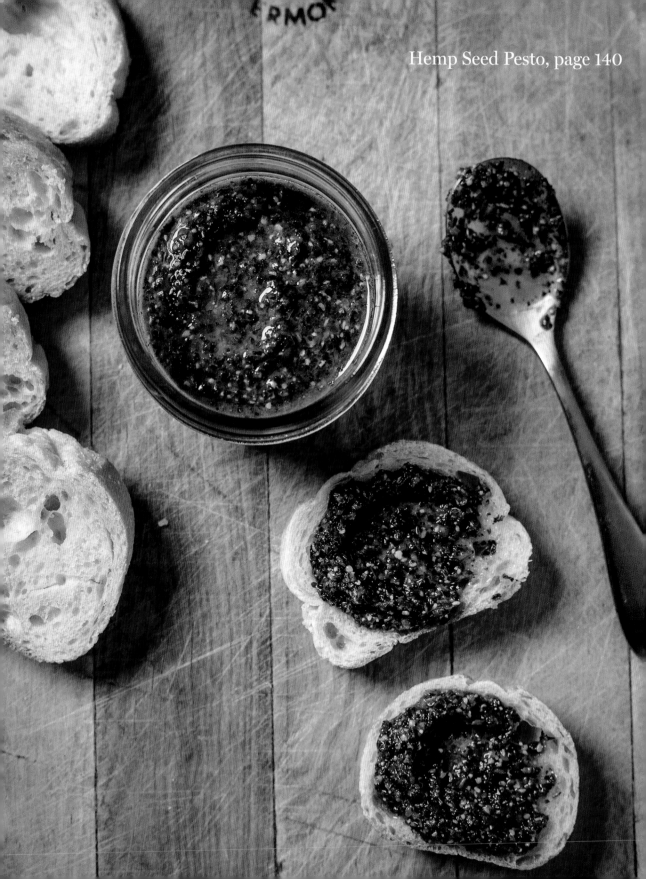

Hemp Seed Pesto, page 140

Salads and Soups

Have you ever wondered why you have those great big salads for lunch that are chock-full of vegetables, but you can't seem to lose weight *and* you're always hungry? Or you have a nice hearty lunch, but are falling asleep a few hours later *and* need a caffeine/sugar pick-me-up?

If this sounds familiar, it's because your meals aren't chemically balanced. That heaping salad may not have enough protein, or may have too many raw vegetables for digestion. That hearty lunch might contain too much animal protein, which saps your body's digestive energy. So what's the answer? Finding *your* balance.

Here are my general protein guidelines for lunch:

Women: 15 to 25 grams of protein
Men: 20 to 35 grams of protein

We find that these guidelines will fuel you through your busy day while keeping energy levels up and supporting your body's repair processes. If you're the type of person who needs a lot of protein, eat a higher-protein breakfast instead of going too heavy with protein at lunch.

Every person is chemically unique. What works for me probably won't work for you. Some people do well with animal protein at lunch, but we find this to be a very small group. If you do great with a burger or chicken, keep eating it! However, to meet their totals, most people do best with the low-reactive forms of vegetarian protein listed below. Are there other forms of vegetarian proteins? Absolutely! But this is our lowest-reactive list. So if you do well with chickpeas, you can test and see how you do with lentils or pinto beans, which are also on the lower end of reactive beans. If you do well with goat cheese, give cow's cheese a shot!

Low-Reactive Vegetarian Sources of Protein
Broccoli: 4 to 5 grams per cup
Kale: 6 grams per 1½ cups
Chickpeas: 5 grams per ½ cup
Rice: 6 grams per cup
Chia seeds: 5 grams per 2 tablespoons

Sunflower seeds: 5 grams per ounce
Pumpkin seeds: 9 grams per ounce
Hemp seeds: 11 grams per 3 tablespoons
Almonds: 8 grams per ounce
Goat cheese: 8 grams per ounce

Cooked vegetables and soups are easier on digestion and those lovely raw vegetables are a great source of enzymes. The average person usually does very well with a 50/50 cooked-to-raw ratio at lunch. For example: Have 2 cups of soup and 2 cups of salad. I have a more sensitive stomach and have always done better with a 75/25 ratio: 75 percent cooked to 25 percent raw. That's my balance. Find your ratio and you won't believe how much energy you will have, how good you will feel, and how flat your stomach is!

Your preferences may change with the seasons, too. In summer months you may be able to get away with a salad and no cooked vegetables, while in winter you may just want to live off of soups and avoid the raw stuff—finding your path and listening to your body is the key. Certain vegetables, like cucumbers, can be really tough to digest at all in winter, but as soon as those temperatures climb into the eighties this little vegetable can be your best friend!

Remembering how we ate generations ago can give us a key as to what we may be doing incorrectly now. Many cultures—from Jewish to Persian, from Mexican to Korean—eat cucumbers with a mix of ginger, chilies, and limes. Adding ginger to aid digestion and chilies for heat helps break down this sometimes problematic food. Our ancestors were on to something! All of the recipes that call for cucumbers in this book mix them with ginger and chili for better digestion.

So what's the takeaway from all of this? See how you feel after lunch. You shouldn't be hungry or look like you have a food baby. You should feel nicely full until several hours later. Enjoy!

Salads

CALAMARI SALAD

I was intimidated by the thought of calamari until I saw it frozen and cleaned. Very easy and quick to prepare!

    1½ lb cleaned calamari rings
    ½ cup carrot cut into matchsticks
    ⅓ cup extra virgin olive oil
    3 tbsp lemon juice
    1 tbsp balsamic vinegar
    1 cup chopped fresh parsley
    2 cloves garlic, minced
    ¼ tsp freshly ground black pepper
    1 small red onion, chopped
    Optional: 2 stalks celery, chopped (see Note)

Bring a large pot of water to a boil. Rinse squid under cold water. Cook squid in boiling water for 60 seconds. Drain in a colander and transfer to a large bowl of cold water to cool for 5 minutes. Drain squid and pat dry.

In a small pot with a steamer basket, steam carrot matchsticks for 2 minutes.

To make dressing, whisk together olive oil, lemon juice, vinegar, parsley, garlic, and pepper in a small bowl.

In a medium bowl, combine squid, carrot, onion, and celery, if using, and toss together. Add dressing and let marinate for at least 30 minutes before serving. Serve chilled or at room temperature.

Note: Celery is a higher-reactive vegetable, but can do very well with people who have heart and blood pressure issues.

Makes 4 to 6 servings

KALE AND ENOKI MUSHROOM SALAD

All of the medicinal mushrooms, like enoki, shiitake, and maitake, are great for fighting cancer, and enoki mushrooms also help to fight HPV. If you need an extra incentive, enoki mushrooms have the texture of pasta! Rice cooking wine is called for in many of the recipes. If you can't find it, no worries! Use white wine with a dash of sea salt.

    2 tbsp extra virgin olive oil

    3 tbsp minced shallots

    4 cloves garlic, minced

    8 cups chopped deveined kale

    2 oz shiitake mushrooms

    2 tbsp rice cooking wine

    2 oz enoki mushrooms

    2 tbsp hemp seeds

Heat olive oil in a large skillet over medium heat. Add shallots and garlic and sauté for 1 minute, stirring frequently. Add kale and shiitake mushrooms and sauté for 2 to 3 minutes; add rice wine and enoki mushrooms and continue cooking for 1 additional minute, until kale is tender. Transfer mixture to serving bowl and sprinkle with hemp seeds.

Makes 4 servings

GRILLED VEGETABLE SALAD

1 lb carrots, quartered lengthwise

2 zucchini, ends trimmed and quartered lengthwise

2 yellow squash, ends trimmed and quartered lengthwise

1 medium head radicchio, cut into 2-inch strips

¾ cup extra virgin olive oil, plus more for oiling the grate

¼ tsp sea salt

1 large red onion, cut into ½-inch-thick slices

¼ cup chopped fresh basil

¼ cup balsamic vinegar

1 clove garlic, minced

½ tsp grated organic orange zest

¼ tsp grated organic lemon zest

1 head frisee, chopped

1 avocado, cut into 1-inch cubes

Special equipment: soaked wooden skewers

Preheat grill for medium heat and lightly oil the grate.

Combine carrots, zucchini, squash, radicchio, ¼ cup olive oil, and sea salt in a large bowl. Mix thoroughly. Thread raw onion and radicchio onto wooden skewers. Transfer oiled vegetables to the preheated grill, along with skewered onion and radicchio. Grill until skewered vegetables are tender, 5 to 7 minutes, and squash and carrots are tender and slightly charred, 10 to 15 minutes. The vegetables can be served in long strips or chopped. Transfer to a large bowl and sprinkle with basil.

Whisk remaining ½ cup olive oil, vinegar, garlic, and orange and lemon zest together in a bowl to make the dressing. Toss vegetables with dressing and let cool.

Serve grilled vegetables over frisee and top with cubed avocado.

Makes 8 servings

WATERMELON CAPRESE

I love putting all of my garden herbs to use; nothing says summer like watermelon and mint.

1 small watermelon (about 4 pounds), peeled and cut into 1-inch cubes

2 tbsp chopped fresh thyme

6 oz goat cheese, rolled into 1-inch balls

1 tbsp extra virgin olive oil

2 tbsp Persian Pomegranate Sauce (page 140)

2 tsp balsamic vinegar

2 tbsp fresh mint cut into ribbons

Arrange watermelon in the bottom of a medium bowl, sprinkle with thyme, and add goat cheese balls. Whisk olive oil, pomegranate sauce, and balsamic vinegar together in a small bowl and drizzle over salad. Top with mint ribbons and serve.

ISRAELI SALAD

Israeli salads vary from family to family. Israelis whose roots are in North Africa, India, and Persia have different interpretations. Variations on the theme are limitless. The Plan version includes brown rice for a hearty, satisfying lunch.

2 medium carrots, grated

½ small beet, peeled and grated

2 cups red leaf lettuce

1 cup cooked brown rice

⅔ cup sunflower seeds

¼ cup finely chopped fresh flat-leaf parsley or cilantro

Optional: 1 cucumber, peeled, seeded, and finely diced

⅓ cup grated hard goat cheese or chèvre

½ tsp grated organic lemon zest

Juice of 1 lemon (2 to 3 tbsp), or to taste

2 to 3 tbsp extra virgin olive oil, or to taste

2 tsp grated peeled fresh ginger

1 tsp crushed red pepper flakes

In a medium serving bowl, mix together carrots, beet, lettuce, rice, sunflower seeds, parsley or cilantro, and cucumber, if using. In a small bowl, whisk cheese, lemon zest and juice, olive oil, ginger, and crushed red pepper flakes. Drizzle dressing over salad and toss. Taste and adjust seasonings as needed.

Note: As this salad contains cucumbers and many raw vegetables, it is best as a summer salad.

Makes 2 to 4 servings

KALE, AVOCADO, AND CRANBERRY SALAD

This is a great dish for everyone, but especially vegans. You can easily meet your lunchtime protein goals and some nice calcium goals, too! A 1½-cup serving of kale will net you 6 grams of protein and 150 milligrams of calcium, and when you add in the sunflower seeds, it's bumped up to 11 grams protein and 200 milligrams calcium!

  2 tbsp extra virgin olive oil
  1 large clove garlic, minced
  8 cups chopped deveined kale
  1 tsp rice vinegar (natural, not seasoned)
  1 avocado, cut into 1-inch cubes
  ¼ cup sunflower seeds
  ⅓ cup dried cranberries
  1 medium carrot, sliced into thin strips
  ⅓ cup raw almonds
  ¼ cup Lime Agave Vinaigrette (page 148)

Heat oil in a large skillet over medium heat. Add garlic and sauté for 30 seconds, then add kale and sauté for an additional 2 minutes, until wilted. Add rice vinegar and stir an additional 30 seconds. Transfer to a medium bowl and let cool. Add avocado, sunflower seeds, cranberries, carrot, and almonds and toss. Drizzle with vinaigrette and serve.

Makes 2 to 4 servings

DELICATA AND KALE SALAD

It's hard to choose a favorite vegetable, but, boy, is delicata squash up there. The sweetness stands up nicely to kale and the colors combine so beautifully. Add some hemp seeds or pumpkin seeds and you have another delectable salad that is dairy-free and high in protein.

    2 tbsp extra virgin olive oil
    1 medium delicata squash, cut into ½-inch cubes
    ¼ cup Carrot Soup Essence (page 102) or vegetable stock
    4 cups chopped deveined kale
    1 green apple, cored and chopped
    Optional: ¼ cup hemp seeds or pumpkin seeds

Heat olive oil in a medium skillet over medium heat. Add squash and sauté for 1 minute. Add soup essence, cover, and cook for 5 minutes, until squash is tender. Add kale and sauté, uncovered, for one additional minute, until kale starts to wilt. Transfer to serving bowl and top with chopped green apple and seeds, if desired.

Makes 2 servings

MOROCCAN CARROT SALAD

I remember the first time I had this delicious, oh-so-simple salad; it was made by friends who own Cafe Mogador in New York City's East Village. I couldn't believe how something so simple could taste so amazing!

    8 medium carrots, cut into ¼-inch-thick slices
    ¼ cup extra virgin olive oil
    4 cloves garlic, crushed
    1 tsp ground cumin
    ½ tsp coriander
    ⅛ tsp sea salt
    1 tsp freshly ground black pepper
    ½ tsp grated organic orange zest
    Juice of ½ lemon (1 to 1½ tbsp)
    Optional: 1 tsp crushed red pepper flakes

Steam carrots in a pot of boiling water for 4 minutes.

Heat olive oil in a large skillet. Add carrots, garlic, cumin, coriander, salt, and pepper. Cook over medium-high heat, stirring and turning carrots, for 4 to 5 minutes, until carrots are tender but not too soft. Add orange zest and sprinkle with lemon juice. Add crushed red pepper flakes, if using. Serve warm or at room temperature.

Makes 4 to 6 servings

RADICCHIO AND POMEGRANATE SALAD

Every time I have people over for dinner I serve this family favorite. People are amazed at how delicious and simple it is! The combination of bitter and sweet is marvelous, and bitter vegetables like radicchio are amazing for gallbladder and liver health.

1 medium head radicchio, chopped
½ cup pomegranate arils
¼ cup salad dressing of choice

Place radicchio in a medium bowl, garnish with pomegranates, and toss with dressing. Serve at room temperature.

Makes 4 to 6 servings

CARROT BEET SALAD

I've been eating a carrot beet salad since my early teens when I first started baking at a hippie health food restaurant. The raw vegetables are pretty easy to digest and chock-full of lovely enzymes. The simple recipe, a standard in naturopathic medicine, aids liver cleansing and is reputed to be strongly anticancer. Adding lemon or lime juice and EVO further helps liver and gallbladder cleansing.

4 large carrots, coarsely grated
1 beet, peeled and coarsely grated
Lime Agave Vinaigrette (page 148) or lemon juice and extra virgin olive oil, to taste

Put all ingredients in a large bowl and toss to combine. Serve immediately.

Makes 4 to 6 servings

ROASTED VEGETABLE, FRISEE,
AND MANCHEGO SALAD

Frisee and all bitter herbs are great for stimulating bile, which aids gallbladder and liver function. That may not sound very sexy, but you'll love the effects!

1 lb carrots, chopped

2 zucchini, chopped

3 cups large broccoli florets

2 large red onions, chopped

6 large shiitake mushrooms, halved

8 cloves garlic, peeled

½ cup extra virgin olive oil

1 tbsp dried rosemary

1 tbsp dried basil

1 tsp dried thyme

½ tsp dried oregano

½ tsp sea salt

1 head frisee, chopped (about 5 cups)

½ cup grated Manchego

Preheat oven to 375°F. Combine carrots, zucchini, broccoli, onion, mushrooms, and garlic with the olive oil and dried herbs and salt in a large bowl. Transfer to a large baking dish and roast for 35 to 40 minutes, until vegetables are tender. Let vegetables cool approximately 30 minutes. Serve on a bed of frisee and top with grated Manchego.

Serves 6 to 8

ORANGE-BASIL CHICKPEA SALAD

Basil and thyme aid digestion—perfect for any bean salad!

    4 cups red leaf or baby lettuce
    2 cups low-sodium chickpeas (100 mg or less per ½-cup serving)
    1 cup grated carrot
    1 avocado, cut into 1-inch cubes
    ¼ cup finely chopped red onion
    ¼ cup coarsely chopped fresh basil
    Orange Thyme Sauce (page 144)

Combine all ingredients in a medium bowl and toss.

    Makes 4 servings

GINGER CUCUMBER SALAD

In Chinese medicine, vegetables like cucumber are considered to be tough to digest raw because they are "cold" and thus hamper digestion. Colder vegetables like cucumber and romaine hearts are best to have in warmer months when our bodies are warmed by the sun. Make sure to have this salad when the mercury hits the eighties!

    ½ cup rice vinegar (natural, not seasoned)
    1 to 2 tbsp chopped peeled fresh ginger
    1 clove garlic, peeled
    1 tsp agave nectar
    2 large cucumbers, seeded and chopped
    ¼ cup sliced red onion
    ¼ cup chopped fresh mint
    ½ tsp grated organic orange zest
    1 to 2 small chili peppers, finely chopped

To make dressing, combine rice vinegar, ginger, garlic, and agave in a food processor. Blend well.

In a medium bowl, combine cucumbers, onion, and mint. Add dressing and orange zest and mix well. Top salad with chopped chilies. Let marinate at least 30 minutes (or up to 48 hours in the fridge).

Makes 4 servings

SPRING SALAD

Spring is a traditional time to clean your liver and gallbladder. Dandelion, apple, and mint can do the trick with this quick and easy salad.

- 4 cups red leaf lettuce
- 2 cups organic dandelion greens, chopped
- 1 apple, cored and cut into 1-inch pieces
- 1 pear, cored and cut into 1-inch pieces
- 1 avocado, cut into 1-inch pieces
- 2 tbsp chopped fresh mint
- Dressing of choice, or a simple dressing of lemon juice and extra virgin olive oil (for extra cleansing effects), to taste

Combine lettuce, dandelion greens, apple, pear, avocado, and mint in medium bowl and toss. Serve with dressing of choice.

Makes 6 servings

ZUCCHINI SLAW

Great for July Fourth BBQ! Dress the salad right before serving to keep it crisp. Best served in summer.

- 2 medium zucchini, coarsely shredded and squeezed dry
- 1 cup grated carrot
- ¼ cup finely chopped onion
- ¼ tsp salt
- 1 tsp freshly ground black pepper
- ½ cup Dairy-Free Ranch Dressing (page 150) or ¼ cup goat cheese

Combine all ingredients in a large bowl and serve immediately.

Makes 6 to 8 servings

WARM DANDELION SALAD

2 tbsp extra virgin olive oil
1 large red onion, chopped
4 cloves garlic, chopped
1 large bunch organic dandelion greens, trimmed and chopped (about 6 cups)
2 tbsp raisins
2 tbsp rice cooking wine
¼ cup hemp seeds

In a large skillet, heat olive oil over medium heat. Add onion and garlic and sauté for 4 minutes, until onion starts to soften. Add dandelion greens and raisins and stir-fry for 2 minutes. Add rice wine and stir an additional minute. Transfer greens to a medium bowl, top with hemp seeds, and serve warm.

Makes 4 to 6 servings

Zucchini Pasta

There are so many ways to make zucchini noodles (completely grain-free noodles that are made just out of zucchini and nothing else) that it boggles the mind, and for many who can't tolerate traditional or gluten-free pasta, it is a godsend! Zucchini is low reactive, inexpensive year-round, easy to grow, and especially plentiful in summer.

It's also a rich source of potassium, which helps the heart and kidneys regulate, and a moderate source of carotene and lutein—essential antioxidants. It is also a moderate source of folates, which are important in cell division and synthesis. Folates are especially important prior to and during pregnancy to help prevent birth defects.

There are many ways to make zucchini pasta, from using a mandolin to using a vegetable peeler. But my easy, lazy way is to use a Paderno spiral vegetable slicer; it runs from $30 to $40. The best part is that this is easy enough for older kids to operate (my eight-year-old uses it).

ZUCCHINI PASTA SALAD

1 tbsp extra virgin olive oil
4 cups zucchini "pasta" (see box)
¼ cup dried cranberries

½ cup almond slivers

4 oz goat cheese, crumbled

Optional: ¼ cup Hemp Seed Pesto (page 140)

Heat olive oil in a large skillet over medium heat. Add zucchini pasta and sauté for 2 to 3 minutes, until slightly softened. Immediately transfer to a large bowl. Add cranberries, almonds, and goat cheese and toss. Drizzle hemp seed pesto on salad, if desired.

Makes 2 to 4 servings

Soups

CARROT GINGER SOUP

Carrot Ginger Soup, a mainstay of *The Plan*, is wonderfully anti-inflammatory and helps to rapidly restore gastrointestinal balance after you eat a reactive food. This recipe, updated from *The Plan*, is for making the soup in bulk. This allows you to take advantage of those 5- and 10-pound bags of carrots on sale, and to save time by freezing the excess for future use!

1 tbsp ground cinnamon

1 tbsp ground cumin

1 tbsp freshly ground black pepper

1 tsp ground cloves

1 tsp cardamom

½ tsp turmeric

½ tsp allspice

7 quarts water

5 lb carrots, chopped

2 large red onions, chopped

3 large zucchini, chopped

8 cloves garlic, peeled

5 to 6 inches fresh ginger, peeled

2 tbsp extra virgin olive oil

Combine cinnamon, cumin, black pepper, cloves, cardamom, turmeric, and allspice in a dry skillet over medium-low heat and cook, stirring constantly, for 30 seconds. In a large soup pot, combine water, carrots, onions, zucchini, garlic, ginger, and olive oil; add toasted spices. Bring water to a boil and then let simmer for 45 minutes, until carrots are soft.

Reserve 2 to 4 quarts of the broth for future soup stocks. Transfer remaining soup to a blender in batches and puree.

Note: Add 1 (14-oz) can of full-fat unsweetened coconut milk and 5 to 6 Vietnamese chili peppers while cooking for a creamier, spicier soup!

Makes 5 quarts (10 to 16 servings)

A Note on Coconut Milk

Canned coconut milk can vary in size from 13.5 to 15.5 ounces per can. The ratio of fat to water varies widely, too. (My favorite brand of coconut milk is called Chaokoh—so rich and creamy!) So obviously these variations will cause differences in batch to batch of your sauces and stews. I wouldn't worry about it. Keep testing different brands and see what works best for your palate. These variations won't change the weight loss and anti-inflammatory effects of the meals, so relax and enjoy!

CARROT SOUP ESSENCE (PLAN VEGAN SOUP STOCK)

This simple soup stock can be used as a starter to soups and sauces or you can use it in lieu of cooking wine for your sautés.

  2 tbsp extra virgin olive oil

  2 cups chopped leeks

  1 large white onion, finely chopped

  3 cloves garlic, minced

  2 tbsp dried sage

  1 tsp freshly ground black pepper

  ½ tsp sea salt

4 quarts broth from Carrot Ginger Soup (page 101) or low-sodium vegetable stock

¼ cup Low-Reactive Tomato Sauce (page 137)

½ cup chopped fresh parsley

1 bay leaf

In a large skillet, heat olive oil over medium heat. Add leeks, onion, garlic, sage, pepper, and salt and sauté for 2 to 3 minutes, until onion is translucent.

In a medium-large soup pot, combine broth, tomato sauce, parsley, and bay leaf and bring to a boil. Add sautéed onion mixture and simmer for 20 minutes. Strain broth through a colander set over a large bowl. Discard solids. Use broth immediately or freeze in batches.

Makes about 16 cups

CREAM OF BROCCOLI SOUP

A protein-rich, delicious, creamy soup that is a family favorite. Feel free to leave out the chilies if you want to tone down the heat.

3 tbsp unsalted butter

1 large onion, chopped

1 tbsp dried sage

1 tsp ground cumin

½ tsp dried celery seed

2 cups low-sodium or homemade chicken stock, vegetable stock, or broth from Carrot Ginger Soup (page 101)

2 cups water

1 (14-oz) can full-fat unsweetened coconut milk

8 cups chopped broccoli (from about 4 heads)

4 cups chopped zucchini (from about 2 medium)

1 small cayenne pepper, or 1 tbsp Sriracha

1 medium avocado, peeled and pitted

In a medium skillet, melt butter over medium heat. Add onion, sage, cumin, and celery seed and sauté until onion is tender. In a medium soup pot, combine sautéed onion, stock or broth, water, coconut milk, broccoli, zucchini, and cayenne pepper or Sriracha. Bring water to a boil and simmer vegetables until tender, about 30 minutes. Transfer soup to blender in batches and blend, adding avocado.

Makes 6 to 8 servings

TOM YUM TALAY

Tom yum is a very popular Thai soup, renowned for its health benefits and ability to fight a cold!

  2 quarts low-sodium or homemade chicken stock, or Carrot Soup Essence (page 102)
  1 small onion, diced
  4 cloves garlic, minced
  2 tbsp grated peeled fresh ginger
  2 to 3 small red Vietnamese chili peppers or 1 to 2 large cayenne peppers, diced very fine
  1 lb scallops, flounder, or halibut
  1 stalk lemongrass, minced
  1 (14-oz) can full-fat unsweetened coconut milk
  1 tbsp agave nectar
  ½ tsp grated organic lime zest
  4 cups zucchini "pasta" (see page 100)
  Juice from 2 limes
  Optional garnishes: ¼ cup chopped basil leaves, 1 cup enoki mushrooms
  Additional seasonings to taste: cumin, kaffir lime leaves, coriander, cinnamon, cilantro

In a medium soup pot over medium heat, combine stock or soup essence, onion, garlic, ginger, and chilies and simmer for 8 to 10 minutes. Add seafood, lemongrass, coconut milk, agave, and lime zest and simmer for 5 minutes. Add zucchini pasta and cook for an additional 2 to 3 minutes. Serve warm, with lime juice and optional garnishes and additional seasonings of choice.

Makes 4 to 6 servings

CHICKPEA VEGETABLE SOUP

The extra cooking time for already-cooked chickpeas makes them easier to digest. So if you found that chickpeas didn't receive a green light when testing, try them in this soup!

1 quart low-sodium or homemade vegetable stock, or Carrot Soup Essence (page 102)

2 cups water

¾ cup Low-Reactive Tomato Sauce (page 137)

1 large white onion, chopped

6 cloves garlic, chopped

1 head kale, deveined and chopped

1 lb carrots, chopped

2 zucchini, chopped, or 5 cups zucchini "pasta" (see page 100)

1 can (16-oz) low-sodium chickpeas (100 milligrams of sodium or less per ½ cup), drained and rinsed

1 tbsp dried sage

1 tbsp dried basil

2 tsp dried rosemary

1 tsp dried oregano

1 tsp freshly ground black pepper

Optional garnish: fresh basil slivers

In a medium soup pot, combine stock and water and bring to a boil. Add remaining ingredients, except for garnish, and let simmer for 40 minutes. Serve warm, garnished with basil if you like.

Makes 4 to 6 servings

CHICKEN STOCK IN A SLOW COOKER

Okay, I admit it, I'm the ultimate, always-cooking home cook, but I never made my own chicken stock on a regular basis until I bought a slow cooker. Save money, get more nutrients and less sodium with this easier than easy recipe! This is a great one to start at night and wake up to in the morning.

3½ quarts water or Carrot Soup Essence (page 102)

8 chicken thighs with skin and bone

2 large red onions, halved

6 large carrots, halved

6 cloves garlic, chopped

1 tbsp honey

2 tbsp dried sage

2 tsp freshly ground black pepper

1 bay leaf

1 tsp sea salt

1 tsp dried thyme

1 tsp ground cumin

Special equipment: 6-quart slow cooker

Place all ingredients in slow cooker, cover, and cook on medium for 6 to 8 hours. Use a slotted spoon to remove the chicken, carrots, and onions (they can be reserved for chicken tostadas or other dishes that call for well-stewed chicken). Place a cheesecloth or coffee filters inside a colander set over a medium pot and strain the stock. Discard the solids. Let stock cool for 20 minutes. Use within 2 days or freeze the stock.

Makes 3 quarts (about 10 servings)

SLOW COOKER CHICKEN "NOODLE" SOUP

Okay, okay. It's not really noodles, but zucchini pasta is a winner in this remake of the classic.

6 cups low-sodium or homemade chicken stock

2 quarts water or Carrot Soup Essence (page 102)

4 chicken thighs with skin and bone, or 2 chicken breasts with skin and bone

2 lb carrots, chopped

1 large red onion, chopped

4 cloves garlic, peeled

2 tbsp dried parsley

1 tbsp dried sage

1 bay leaf

1 head kale, deveined and chopped

4 cups zucchini "pasta" (see page 100)

6 shiitake or enoki mushrooms

Optional garnish: dried or fresh herbs of choice

Special equipment: 6-quart slow cooker

In the slow cooker, combine stock, water or soup essence, chicken, carrots, onion, garlic, parsley, sage, and bay leaf. Cover and cook on high for 6 hours. In the last 30 minutes, add kale, zucchini pasta, and mushrooms. Serve hot or warm, garnished with herbs of your choice, as desired.

Makes 8 to 10 servings

SOPA DE LIMA

You can find Mexican oregano in specialty spice stores, online, and in Mexican grocery stores.

2 tbsp extra virgin olive oil

1 medium onion, chopped

3 carrots, chopped

1 jalapeño pepper, stemmed, seeded, and finely chopped

4 cloves garlic, finely chopped

1 bay leaf

½ tsp dried oregano or Mexican oregano

½ cup Low-Reactive Tomato Sauce (page 137)

4 cups Carrot Soup Essence (page 102) or water

4 cups low-sodium or homemade chicken stock

1 lb chicken thighs, with skin and bone

2 scallions, chopped

Juice of 2 limes (about ¼ cup)

Optional garnish: ¼ cup minced fresh parsley (low reactive) or ¼ cup minced fresh cilantro (moderate low reactive), individual lime wedges

Optional garnish: crumbled Veg Chia Crisps (page 120)

Heat oil in a medium skillet over medium heat. Add onion, carrots, and jalapeño and cook until onion is soft, 4 to 5 minutes. Add garlic, bay leaf, and oregano and cook, stirring, for 1 minute.

In a medium soup pot, combine tomato sauce, soup essence or water, stock, and cooked onion/carrot mixture and bring to a boil. Add chicken and simmer for 25 to 30 minutes.

Let soup cool for 10 minutes and remove the chicken. Shred chicken from bone and add back to soup pot with scallions and lime juice. Simmer and stir for 2 minutes. Discard bay leaf. Serve immediately, garnished with parsley or cilantro, lime wedges, and crumbled crackers, if you like.

Makes 6 to 8 servings

SPROUTED LENTIL SOUP

Celery is a test for most, but tends to do very well with people who have high or low blood pressure or heart conditions. Store-bought dried sprouted lentils are a boon to the time-pressed because they cook in 5 minutes. You can find them at health food stores and online. Sprouting beans makes them more digestible and that means more health benefits and better weight loss.

  2 tbsp extra virgin olive oil
  1 small red onion, chopped
  1 lb carrots, chopped
  1 cup chopped deveined kale or ½ cup chopped celery
  3 cloves garlic, chopped
  ½ cup Low-Reactive Tomato Sauce (page 137)
  2 quarts vegetarian stock or Carrot Soup Essence (page 102)
  2 cups store-bought dried sprouted lentils

Heat oil in a soup pot over medium heat. Add onion, carrots, and kale or celery and sauté for 3 to 4 minutes. Add garlic and sauté for 1 additional minute. Add tomato sauce, stock or soup essence, and sprouted lentils. Cook until lentils are tender, about 5 minutes.

Makes 4 servings

VEGAN CREAM OF MUSHROOM SOUP

2 tbsp extra virgin olive oil

½ yellow onion, diced

1½ cups diced mixed shiitake and enoki mushrooms

1 tsp onion powder

¼ tsp sea salt

Freshly ground black pepper, to taste

1 cup Carrot Soup Essence (page 102)

2 cups canned full-fat unsweetened coconut milk

In a medium skillet, heat oil over medium heat. Add onion and sauté 4 minutes. Add mushrooms, onion powder, salt, and pepper. Reduce heat to medium low and cook an additional minute, stirring frequently. Add soup essence, reduce the heat to low, and cook for 5 minutes more. Add coconut milk and stir for 1 minute. Serve immediately.

Makes 2 servings

HEARTY TOMATO BASIL SOUP

This is the soup that I serve to my clients when they test Low-Reactive Tomato Sauce (page 137) for the first time! Feel free to add more tomato sauce and pesto to bump up the flavors.

2 tbsp extra virgin olive oil

1 medium onion, chopped

4 cloves garlic, finely chopped

¼ cup Hemp Seed Pesto (page 140)

1 cup Low-Reactive Tomato Sauce (page 137)

1 cup Carrot Soup Essence (page 102) or water

2 cups low-sodium or homemade chicken stock

1 lb chicken thighs, skinned, deboned, and chopped

1 lb carrots, chopped

2 blue potatoes, chopped

Heat the oil in a medium skillet over medium heat. Add onion and garlic and sauté for 4 to 5 minutes. Add hemp seed pesto and tomato sauce and cook, stirring, for 1 minute.

In a medium soup pot, combine tomato/onion mixture, soup essence or water, stock, chicken, carrots, and potatoes and simmer for 25 to 30 minutes, until chicken is thoroughly cooked. Serve immediately.

Makes 6 to 8 servings

CHAPTER 8

Side Dishes and Appetizers

Balancing raw and cooked vegetables is essential to optimal digestion, as you now know, and a diverse selection of small dishes can ensure that you are getting a variety of foods to maximize nutrition and satiation. It's also a wonderful way to try new foods and spices—think of these recipes as your very own tapas restaurant!

Included in this section are a few items that can be reactive when eaten in large amounts, such as Brussels sprouts, tomato sauce, and potatoes. But these are very friendly when combined with other vegetables and eaten in small amounts, So if you've tested these foods on their own and they haven't been your best friend, try them in these recipes. It's also important to remember to keep retesting foods that didn't work for you before. Giving your body a rest from mildly reactive foods usually means you can enjoy them on occasion after a few months of abstinence.

Just in case you were wondering if having a variety of colors on your dinner plate means you are getting optimal nutrition, the answer is yes! Red and orange vegetables usually have the highest vitamin C and are rich sources of vitamin A and lycopene, both of which are powerful antioxidants. Green vegetables are usually the most nutrient dense and are often rich in iron. Blue and purple foods contain a powerful antioxidant, anthocyanin, which protects against heart disease and cancer. Red foods like beets contain betalains which provide antioxidant, anti-inflammatory, and detoxification support. The list goes on with the wonderful, health-supporting ways in which food is in fact, your medicine. So brighten up that plate with some of these quick and easy dishes.

PLAN HUMMUS

Our Plan hummus does not contain tahini, but it's just as delicious as the traditional recipe, and much less reactive!

    2 cups low-sodium chickpeas, drained and rinsed
    ½ cup extra virgin olive oil, plus additional for drizzling
    Juice of 1 lemon (about 3 tbsp)
    2 tbsp water
    2 cloves garlic, peeled
    2 tsp ground cumin, to taste, plus a sprinkling for garnish
    ⅛ tsp sea salt
    Freshly ground black pepper, to taste
    Optional garnish: chopped fresh parsley leaves, fresh dill, or fresh chives

Combine all ingredients, except for garnish, in a food processor and blend for 1 minute. Taste and adjust seasoning (you may want to add more lemon juice). To serve, drizzle with additional olive oil and sprinkle with a bit more cumin and some parsley, dill, or chives, if desired. Serve immediately or refrigerate up to 5 days.

Makes 7 to 8 servings (about 2 cups)

ZUCCHINI SALSA

For our friends who have a hard time with tomatoes, zucchini is another gift of summer and an alternative salsa vegetable that is high in potassium. If you have a hard time digesting raw zucchini, try roasting it prior to prep.

    1 large zucchini, cut into ½-in cubes (about 2 cups)
    1 medium red onion, finely chopped
    Juice of 2 limes (about 3 tbsp)
    2 cloves garlic, finely chopped
    1 jalapeño pepper, stemmed, seeded, and chopped
    Sea salt and freshly ground black pepper, to taste
    Optional: ¼ cup chopped fresh cilantro

Combine all ingredients in a small bowl. Serve immediately or refrigerate for up to 3 days.

Makes 4 servings (about 2 cups)

PLAN GUACAMOLE

2 ripe avocados, halved and pitted
½ red onion, minced
Juice of ½ lime (about 1 tbsp)
2 tbsp water
⅛ tsp sea salt
Freshly ground black pepper
Optional: ½ tsp chipotle powder or ½ tsp roasted jalapeños, diced

Place avocado in a medium bowl (reserve pits if not serving immediately). Using a fork, mash avocado. Add onion, lime juice, water, salt, pepper, and chipotle powder or jalapeños, if using, and continue to blend.

Serve immediately or place pits back in guacamole mix to keep it from turning brown.

Makes 4 to 6 servings (about 2 cups)

5-LAYER DIP

Our 5-layer dip is a big hit at Super Bowl parties and brunches. Serve with your favorite chips.

2 cups Plan Hummus (page 113)
4 oz goat-cheese ricotta
1 cup Zucchini Salsa (page 113)
2 cups Plan Guacamole (above)
4 oz grated goat-cheese Gouda
Optional garnish: black olives

Layer ingredients in a glass pie dish or baking pan as follows: hummus, ricotta, salsa, guacamole, and finish with Gouda. Top with olives, if you like.

Makes 8 to 10 servings

HEMP SEED HUMMUS

8 cloves garlic, peeled

1 medium to large zucchini, chopped

⅓ cup hemp seeds

2 tbsp sunflower seeds

2 tbsp lemon juice

1 tbsp extra virgin olive oil

1 tbsp dried rosemary

⅛ tsp sea salt

2 tbsp water

Optional: ¼ tsp grated organic lemon or organic orange zest

Preheat oven to 300°F. Place garlic in a small roasting dish and roast for 40 minutes, until cloves are soft to the touch. Combine roasted garlic, zucchini, hemp seeds, sunflower seeds, lemon juice, olive oil, rosemary, salt, and water in a food processor and blend for 1 minute. Transfer to a serving bowl and top with zest, if desired.

Makes 4 servings (about 1½ cups)

ROASTED NUTS

Roasted nuts are delicious and may actually be easier to digest for some folks. The problem with store-bought nuts is that they are usually roasted with oils like cottonseed oil, which is high in saturated fats and pesticides (yum?). And they are often roasted at too high a temperature, which degrades oils, and then can lie around on the shelves, which can make their oils rancid. Rancid oils attract free radicals, which means your healthy nut has turned into a high-inflammatory snack. You can easily take care of this (and save money) by roasting your own nuts!

1 lb any nut or seed of your choosing

Preheat oven to 250°F. Place nuts or seeds on a baking sheet and roast for 20 minutes. Let cool. Store in airtight container for up to 1 week.

SPICY EXTRA VIRGIN OLIVE OIL DIP

Zeytinyagi is a Turkish dipping sauce that is amazing with bread fresh out of the oven. Remember fats slow down the absorption of sugars, so try to always have your bread with a little extra virgin olive oil or butter.

½ tsp dried mint

½ tsp freshly ground black pepper

¼ tsp thyme

¼ tsp ground cumin

⅛ tsp sea salt

¼ tsp grated organic lemon or organic orange zest

½ cup extra virgin olive oil

In a dry small saucepan, toast mint, pepper, thyme, and cumin over low heat until fragrant. Combine toasted spices with salt, zest, and olive oil in a small serving bowl and let sit for 30 to 60 minutes. The dip is good for up to 5 days. Serve with warm bread of choice.

Makes 4 servings (½ cup)

CREAMED KALE DIP

Delicious for crudités, crackers, or as a sandwich spread.

1 bunch kale, deveined and roughly chopped

1 small red onion, chopped

2 cloves garlic, chopped

2 tbsp extra virgin olive oil

2 tbsp low-sodium or homemade chicken or vegetable stock

1 cup goat-cheese ricotta

2 tbsp grated Manchego

1 tsp onion powder

In a large saucepan, combine kale, onion, garlic, and olive oil and cook over medium heat for 2 minutes. Add stock, cover, and cook for an additional 8 to 10 minutes, until kale is soft. Transfer kale mixture to a food processor and add ricotta, Manchego, and onion powder. Blend for 1 to 2 minutes, until mixture is creamy and chunky. Serve immediately or refrigerate for up to 4 days.

Makes 4 servings (about 1½ cups)

GOAT CHEESE TRIO

Lavender, Chamomile, and Honey ~ Orange and Black Pepper ~ Rosemary and Garlic

This simple and elegant dish is one of my favorite appetizers to serve at summer parties. I just see what's growing in my garden and is ready to harvest. Feel free to improvise with your garden's or greenmarket's bounty.

1 (10-oz) log goat cheese

Lavender, Chamomile, and Honey

1 tsp dried or fresh lavender

½ tsp dried chamomile flowers

1 tsp honey or agave nectar

Orange and Black Pepper

1 tsp grated organic orange zest

1 tsp coarse ground pepper

Rosemary and Garlic

1 tbsp fresh rosemary

1 tsp garlic powder

Divide the goat cheese log into 15 pieces and form into balls or discs. Place the herb mixes into each of 3 small ramekins (do not mix seasonings). Roll each cheese ball in one dish and place on a serving plate. Refrigerate for 15 to 20 minutes to chill and then serve.

Makes 6 servings

SHIITAKE PÂTÉ

One of my fave party appetizers, it's delicious on a warm baguette. Try not to eat the whole bowl before the party starts!

  2 tbsp extra virgin olive oil

  3 cups shiitake mushrooms, chopped

  2 tbsp sunflower seeds

  Dash of sea salt

  Optional: 2 tbsp truffle oil

Heat olive oil in a medium sauté pan over medium heat. Add shiitakes and cook, stirring as juices are released. Turn heat down to medium low so juices don't escape, and sauté 4 to 5 minutes longer, until shiitakes are soft. Transfer shiitakes and their juice to a food processor, add sunflower seeds, and blend. Season with salt. If you like, stir in truffle oil for truffle flavor, or add additional extra virgin olive oil.

Makes 8 to 10 servings

ROSEMARY–BLACK PEPPER POTATO CHIPS

I missed the incredible salt-free potato chips from Trader Joe's when they were discontinued. So I started to make my own, and now you can, too!

  2 medium potatoes

  ¼ cup extra virgin olive oil

  1 tbsp dried rosemary, crumbled

  2 tsp freshly ground black pepper

  Optional: ¼ cup grated Parmesan

Slice potatoes on a mandolin or a food processor as thin as you can; I like them ⅛ inch thick. If you can, soak potatoes in about 4 cups water for 20 minutes to remove starch. Pat dry.

Preheat oven to 375°F. In a medium bowl, liberally coat potatoes with the olive oil, rosemary, and pepper. Arrange potatoes on a baking sheet without overlapping. Bake for 18 to 20 minutes, removing chips as they brown. If you like, sprinkle Parmesan on chips as they come out of the oven.

Makes 4 servings

KATIE'S KALE CHIPS

These chips are named after our very own Dr. Katie; they're a great way to introduce people to kale. I wish they would keep longer but they are so delicious they don't last long at our house!

1 head kale, rinsed, deveined, fully dried, and chopped
1 tbsp extra virgin olive oil
Pinch of sea salt
Freshly ground black pepper
Optional: 1 tbsp garlic powder
Fresh lime juice

Preheat oven to 120°F. Make sure kale is dry. Coat kale lightly with olive oil and then season with salt, pepper, and garlic powder, if using. Spread out on baking sheets and bake for 40 to 60 minutes, until crispy. Let cool, sprinkle with lime juice and enjoy immediately.

Makes 2 to 3 servings

APPLE CUMIN CHIPS

2 medium Granny Smith apples, cored
2 tsp ground cumin
1 tsp ground cinnamon
Dash of sea salt

Preheat oven to 200°F. Line a baking sheet with parchment paper.

Slice apples ⅛ inch thick on a mandolin or in a food processor. Combine cumin, cinnamon, and salt in a ramekin. Arrange apple slices on prepared baking sheet in a single layer without overlapping and sprinkle with spice mix.

Bake apple chips for 60 minutes. Flip to the other side and bake an additional 40 to 50 minutes, until crispy. Serve warm or let cool. Store in an airtight container for up to 5 days.

Makes 4 servings

VEG CHIA CRISPS

Simple, inexpensive gluten-free crackers that are chock-full of protein!

Carrot Crackers
2 cups grated carrots
⅛ cup whole flaxseeds
⅜ cup chia seeds

Beet Crackers
2 cups grated beets
⅛ cup whole flaxseeds
⅜ cup chia seeds

Olive oil for baking sheets

For the carrot crackers, place ingredients in a food processor and blend, scraping down the sides to get all ingredients incorporated. Form into a ball and let sit for 45 minutes for mucilage to form to bind the ingredients. Repeat with the beet cracker ingredients.

Preheat oven to 225°F. Grease 2 baking sheets with olive oil.

Place carrot dough between 2 sheets of wax paper. Use a rolling pin to roll out dough until it is ⅛ inch thick. Using a 4-inch round cookie cutter, cut out about 8 crackers. Place crackers on prepared sheet. Repeat with beet dough.

Bake crackers for 50 minutes. Flip crackers and bake for an additional 50 minutes, until completely firm. For extra crispy crackers, turn off oven and leave crackers in for 2 to 3 hours.

Makes 6 servings (16 to 18 crackers)

AVOCADO FRIES WITH SWEET 'N' SOUR SAUCE

Fried avocados: as delicious as you'd imagine they are.

   2 tbsp extra virgin olive oil

   2 firm, ripe avocados, halved and pitted

   ½ cup all-purpose flour

   2 large egg whites, beaten

   1½ cups panko bread crumbs

   1 tsp garlic powder

   1 tsp onion powder

   Sweet 'n' Sour Sauce (page 143)

Preheat oven to 425°F. Grease a baking pan with olive oil.

Slice each avocado half into 5 slices and set aside. Set out three shallow bowls: place flour in the first bowl, egg whites in the second, and in the third bowl combine panko, garlic powder, and onion powder. Coat each avocado slice in flour, then egg, and then panko mix. Place avocado fries on prepared pan. Bake for 20 minutes, until the fries are browned. Serve with dipping sauce.

Makes 3 to 4 servings

FLOUR TORTILLAS

Warm flour tortillas are an absolute joy and so easy to make. Store-bought versions and wraps are loaded with chemicals, so try this simple recipe, where coconut oil is used instead of the traditional lard.

   4 cups all-purpose flour

   1½ tsp baking powder

   2 tbsp solidified coconut oil or solidified duck fat

   1½ cups water

   2 tbsp extra virgin olive oil, plus more as needed

In a large mixing bowl, combine flour and baking powder. Mix thoroughly. Slowly add coconut oil or duck fat in batches, until flour is crumbly. Add water and mix thoroughly.

Form into a ball and then roll out on a floured surface. Use a 6-inch cookie cutter to cut out 10 to 12 rounds.

Heat the olive oil in a large skillet over medium heat. Add 2 to 3 tortillas and fry on one side until the tortilla starts to bubble, about 1 minute. Flip and cook an additional 45 to 60 seconds, until lightly browned. Repeat to fry the remaining tortillas, adding additional oil as needed and placing the tortillas in a tortilla warmer to keep warm (or serve as soon as they are finished frying).

Makes 10 to 12 tortillas

SAUTÉED SAVOY CABBAGE WITH GINGER DRESSING

Savoy cabbage is moderate reactive but is a great test for the whole cabbage family, so try this gateway vegetable and see how you feel!

    2 tbsp extra virgin olive oil
    1 medium head Savoy cabbage, cut into 1-inch strips
    6 shiitake mushrooms, chopped
    3 carrots, julienned
    2 tbsp rice cooking wine
    Ginger Dressing (page 138)

In a medium sauté pan, heat olive oil over medium heat. Add cabbage, shiitakes, and carrots and sauté for 2 minutes. Add rice wine and cook for an additional 4 to 5 minutes, until vegetables are tender. Serve warm with Ginger Dressing.

Makes 6 to 8 servings

BAKED RADICCHIO WITH BALSAMIC GLAZE
AND GOAT CHEESE

I can't get enough of radicchio, more bitter than frisee and packing a punch of taste and health. Soaking radicchio keeps the leaves from getting too crispy when baked.

1 head radicchio, ends trimmed, cut into 1-inch-thick slices

1 cup vegetarian stock or Carrot Soup Essence (page 102)

¼ cup balsamic vinegar

2 tbsp honey or agave nectar

4 oz goat cheese

Place radicchio in a shallow baking pan and cover with stock or soup essence. Mix well. Soak for at least 1 hour or let refrigerate overnight.

Preheat oven to 400°F. Drain radicchio and discard stock. In a small saucepan over low heat, combine balsamic vinegar and agave nectar and reduce for 3 to 4 minutes, to about ¼ cup. Drizzle over radicchio. Bake for 12 to 15 minutes, until lightly browned. Top with goat cheese before serving.

Makes 4 servings

BALSAMIC-GRILLED RADICCHIO WITH SHAVED PECORINO

Grilling radicchio gives it a smoky flavor that can't be beat.

⅓ cup extra virgin olive oil, plus more for oiling the grate

2 tbsp balsamic vinegar

3 cloves garlic, chopped

½ tbsp chopped fresh rosemary

½ tsp packed finely grated organic orange zest

½ tsp crushed red pepper flakes

2 large heads radicchio, each quartered through core end

Sea salt and freshly ground black pepper, to taste

¼ cup Pecorino Romano cheese shavings

Whisk together olive oil, vinegar, garlic, rosemary, orange zest, and crushed red pepper flakes in a large bowl. Add radicchio and toss to coat. Let marinate for 15 minutes.

Preheat grill for medium heat and lightly oil the grate. Drain marinade into a small bowl. Place radicchio on grill pan and sprinkle with salt and pepper. Grill radicchio, turning occasionally, until the edges are crisp and slightly charred, about 6 minutes. Transfer radicchio to a serving platter. Drizzle with reserved marinade and sprinkle with cheese shavings.

Makes 8 servings

PANKO-CRUSTED BRUSSELS SPROUTS

Cooking the Brussels sprouts prior to baking helps to deactivate the goitrogens and make them easier to digest!

    1 lb Brussels sprouts, trimmed, halved through the stem end
    5 tbsp extra virgin olive oil
    2 tbsp herbes de Provence or Italian herb blend
    1 cup panko bread crumbs or gluten-free panko
    1 cup chopped leeks
    1 cup chopped carrots
    1 cup finely chopped deveined kale

Preheat oven to 400°F.

Cook Brussels sprouts in a large pot of boiling water for about 5 minutes. Transfer to a large bowl. Combine 3 tbsp olive oil with herbs and pour over Brussels sprouts, turning to coat well. Stir in ¾ cup of the panko.

Place leeks on the bottom of a medium cast-iron skillet and then layer with carrots and kale and top with Brussels sprouts. Sprinkle with remaining ¼ cup panko and drizzle remaining 2 tbsp oil on top. Bake for 18 to 20 minutes, until panko is browned.

Makes 4 servings

PUMPKIN CASSEROLE

A perfect side dish for your winter evenings when pumpkins are in season.

    ¼ cup (½ stick) unsalted butter, softened, plus more for greasing
    4 cups canned or cooked pureed pumpkin, at room temperature

2 large eggs

¼ cup agave nectar

¼ cup Silk coconut milk or Rice Dream

1 tsp pure vanilla extract

1 tsp ground cinnamon

½ tsp allspice

¼ cup nuts of choice

Preheat oven to 375°F. Butter a 9x9-inch casserole dish.

Combine pumpkin, eggs, agave, coconut milk or Rice Dream, ¼ cup butter, vanilla, cinnamon, and allspice in a food processor and blend. Transfer mixture to prepared casserole dish. Bake for 25 to 30 minutes, until browned. Top with nuts of choice.

Makes 8 servings

VEGETABLE TIMBALE

1 large zucchini

1 red onion, peeled

3 cups kale, deveined

2 large carrots

8 shiitake mushrooms

4 to 6 oz soft goat cheese, crumbled

2 oz Parmesan or Manchego, grated

Preheat oven to 400°F.

Use a mandolin to slice zucchini, onion, kale, carrots, and mushrooms as thinly as you can. In an ungreased 9-inch baking dish, create layers as for lasagna, layering vegetables and goat cheese in this order: zucchini, onion, kale, goat cheese, carrots, and shiitakes, then top with Parmesan or Manchego. Bake for 30 minutes, until cheese on top is slightly golden.

Makes 6 servings

GRILLED ZUCCHINI PESTO "SUSHI"

¼ cup extra virgin olive oil, plus more for oiling the grate

4 zucchini

1 cup Hemp Seed Pesto (page 140) or Lemon Sunflower Pesto (page 140)

½ cup cooked basmati rice

1 tbsp chia seeds

Optional: chopped fresh summer herbs of choice such as chives, cilantro, basil, parsley

Preheat grill to 400°F and lightly oil the grate.

Cut off zucchini ends and slice lengthwise on a mandolin into long ¼-inch-thick strips. In a medium bowl, combine zucchini with ¼ cup olive oil to coat liberally. Grill zucchini strips until browned on each side, about 2 minutes. Let cool slightly.

Mix pesto, rice, and chia in a small bowl. Spoon about 1 tablespoon pesto mixture onto one end of a zucchini strip. Roll up strip to make "sushi." Repeat with remaining zucchini strips and pesto mixture. Sprinkle with fresh herbs of choice, if desired, and serve warm.

Makes 8 servings

ROASTED VEGETABLES

This recipe is a great way to test potatoes; they usually work well in small amounts when mixed with other vegetables. To test potatoes, add in 1 medium potato, cut into 1-inch chunks, before baking. Leave out the potato if you are doing the cleanse.

3 large carrots, sliced

1 large zucchini, cut into ½-inch chunks

1 red onion, cut into large chunks

1 head broccoli, cut into 2-inch florets

4 to 5 cloves garlic, peeled

3 tbsp extra virgin olive oil

Fresh or dried Italian herb blend or herbes de Provence, to taste

Sea salt and freshly ground black pepper, to taste

Preheat oven to 375°F.

In a large bowl, toss vegetables and garlic with oil, herbs, salt, and pepper. Transfer to large baking sheet and bake for 35 minutes, until browned.

Makes 8 servings

KOREAN CUCUMBER KIMCHI (*OI SEBAGI*)

Oi Sebagi is a great side dish and wonderful on fish or a burger! Cucumber kimchi is not fermented as so many kimchis are, so you can delight in your efforts right away.

6 Kirby cucumbers, cut into ½-inch cubes

3 stalks Korean flower chives (buchu) or 2 scallions, chopped

3 tbsp Sriracha or gochujang (more reactive)

2 tsp minced garlic

1 tsp grated peeled fresh ginger

⅛ tsp fish sauce

Combine all ingredients in a small mixing bowl. Cover and let marinate 30 minutes or up to 24 hours. Store in an airtight container and use within 4 to 5 days.

JALAPEÑO POPPERS

15 jalapeño peppers (see Note)

8 oz goat cheese

6 oz goat-cheese Gouda, grated

½ cup all-purpose flour

1 tsp garlic powder

1 tsp onion powder

½ cup unsweetened Silk coconut milk or unsweetened Rice Dream

½ cup panko bread crumbs

2 cups grape-seed oil

Optional: Dairy-Free Ranch Dressing (page 150) and/or Chipotle-Avo Dressing (page 151)

Slice jalapeños in half lengthwise. For mild poppers, use a spoon to remove the pith and seeds. If you want some fire, only remove half. In a small bowl, combine both goat cheeses. Spoon cheese mixture into each jalapeño.

In a shallow bowl, combine flour, garlic, and onion powder. Mix well. Dip each stuffed jalapeño into seasoned flour. Let peppers dry for 10 minutes. (If you omit this step the coating will just fall off!)

Place coconut milk or Rice Dream and panko in two separate bowls. Dip peppers into coconut milk or Rice Dream and immediately into panko to coat. Place on a rack. Repeat to coat all peppers. Repeat a second time for extra crispy poppers!

Heat oil in a medium skillet over medium-high heat for 2 minutes. Carefully add 4 or 5 poppers at a time and fry 2 minutes on each side, until browned and tender. Remove with tongs and drain on a paper towel on a plate. Serve with Dairy-Free Ranch Dressing and/or Chipotle-Avo Dressing, if you like.

Note: You may want to wear kitchen gloves when handling jalapeños, they pack a punch!

Makes 8 to 10 servings

CRAB CAKES

¼ cup Plan Guacamole (page 114)

¼ cup store-bought mayonnaise or Aioli (page 143)

¼ cup chopped fresh chives

1 large egg

1 tsp dried tarragon

½ tsp black pepper

1 lb canned or cooked crabmeat, picked through for shells

1 cup panko bread crumbs or gluten-free panko

¼ cup extra virgin olive oil

In a large bowl, whisk together guacamole, mayonnaise or aioli, chives, egg, tarragon, and pepper. Add crab and ½ cup of panko and mix thoroughly to combine. Form mixture into 8 patties. Spread remaining ½ cup panko in a shallow bowl. Coat patties with panko.

Heat oil in a large skillet over medium-high heat. Add the crab cakes and cook until each side is browned, about 3 to 4 minutes per side. Alternatively, you can bake the crab cakes at 475°F for 15 minutes.

Makes 8 mini crab cakes (about 4 servings)

GRILLED TURMERIC CHICKEN WINGS

1 cup canned full-fat unsweetened coconut milk

3 shallots, chopped

3 cloves garlic, peeled

2 jalapeño peppers, stemmed

1 (1-inch) piece fresh ginger, peeled and grated (about ½ tbsp)

2 tbsp fresh lime juice (1 to 1½ limes)

1 tbsp turmeric

1 tsp sea salt

1 cup water

3 lb whole chicken wings

Extra virgin olive oil, for oiling the grate

Lime wedges

Optional: Dairy-Free Ranch Dressing (page 150) for dipping

Combine coconut milk, shallots, garlic, jalapeños, ginger, lime juice, turmeric, salt, and water in a blender. Puree until a smooth marinade forms. Place chicken wings in a large baking dish. Pour marinade over chicken wings, turning to coat evenly. Cover chicken and refrigerate overnight.

Remove chicken from marinade, shaking any excess marinade back into dish. Transfer chicken to a large platter. Let stand at room temperature for 15 minutes.

Preheat grill for medium heat and lightly oil the grate.

Transfer marinade from dish into a large saucepan and bring to a boil over medium heat. Reduce heat to medium low and simmer, stirring occasionally, until marinade thickens, 10 to 15 minutes. Pour half of marinade into a small bowl; set aside for basting chicken while it grills. Keep remaining marinade in saucepan; cover and keep warm until ready to serve with chicken.

Grill chicken wings, turning every 5 minutes and basting occasionally with marinade in small bowl, until fat is rendered, 30 to 35 minutes. (The key here is to turn the wings often so the skin doesn't char or burn.) Continue grilling chicken without basting until wings are cooked through, about 10 minutes longer.

Transfer chicken to a large platter and serve with lime wedges. Transfer warm marinade from saucepan to a small bowl and serve alongside as a dipping sauce. You can also serve with our Dairy-Free Ranch Dressing!

Makes 6 to 8 servings

CHAPTER 9

Sauces and Dressings

Sauces and dressings do so much more than make the same old chicken and zucchini taste like a gourmet meal. They are a way to promote *healing,* and that's what excites me! Having delicious dynamic food that can promote health is what The Plan is all about.

Since time began, we have used herbs, spices, and other seasonings for their culinary benefits as well as their health properties. Below are a few of my favorites and ones that I always have in my kitchen. The recipes throughout this book—but especially in this chapter—draw from all of these high-powered, nutrient-rich herbs and spices. The spices listed are meant to be used for pairing with your food, and not as supplements.

- **Basil** contains vitamin A, vitamin K, vitamin C, magnesium, iron, potassium, and calcium. It's rich in antioxidants and is anti-inflammatory. It aids digestion, helps headaches, and is antibacterial.
- **Black pepper** contains potassium, calcium, zinc, manganese, iron, and magnesium. It is anti-inflammatory, aids digestion, is a mild diuretic, has antibacterial properties, increases stomach acid secretion (which is great if you have low stomach acid), increases absorption of nutrients like selenium, and helps to detoxify the liver.
- **Cardamom** contains potassium, magnesium, and calcium. It is used to relieve digestive complaints like intestinal gas and constipation and for healing kidney, lung, liver, and gallbladder complaints.
- **Cayenne** contains potassium, calcium, beta-carotene, vitamins A, B-complex, C, and E. The capsaicin in cayenne creates heat and healing benefits. It also helps to offset the inflammation that is typically associated with peppers and the nightshade family of vegetables. Cayenne aids digestion, improves circulation, aids weight loss, and removes toxins. Capsaicin creams can be used topically for joint pain and back pain.
- **Cinnamon** contains antioxidants, manganese, fiber, and calcium. It is used to control blood sugar, lower cholesterol, fight yeast, improve circulation, and relieve digestive disorders such as IBS and ulcers. It is also antibacterial and antimicrobial.
- **Cumin** contains antioxidants, iron, calcium, and magnesium. It can aid in the normalization of blood sugar and digestion and is good for lung function and healthy cholesterol levels. It is being studied for its effects on pancreatic enzymes and its anticancer benefits.

- **Garlic** contains selenium and allicin, a sulfur compound that aids iron absorption. It is used for high blood pressure, high cholesterol, aiding immune function, treating bacterial and fungal infections, and aiding lung and liver function.
- **Ginger** aids digestion and glycemic control and diabetes, helps nausea and motion sickness, and reduces inflammation.
- **Lemon zest** contains calcium, vitamin C, and potassium. It reduces cholesterol, strengthens capillaries, cleanses the liver, is anti-inflammatory, and helps to fight skin, breast, and colon cancer. It is best to use organic as pesticides adhere to the oil of citrus skin.
- **Onion** contains quercetin, a strong anti-inflammatory oxidant. It also has vitamin C and chromium, which controls blood sugar. It also lowers blood pressure, lowers cholesterol, and is anticancer.
- **Orange zest** contains beta carotene, potassium, pectin, and vitamin C. It helps normalize blood sugar and lower cholesterol, plus it's anti-inflammatory and fights skin, breast, and colon cancer. It is best to use organic as pesticides adhere to the oil of citrus skin.
- **Rosemary** contains calcium, vitamin A, vitamin C, iron, pantothenic acid, and folic acid. It reduces inflammation, helps arthritic pain, stimulates the immune system, and improves digestion and circulation.
- **Sage** contains vitamin A, vitamin B6, iron, and magnesium. It aids lung function and has antibacterial and antiseptic properties. When eaten or consumed as a tea, it is useful for helping combat night sweats. It is also great to use as a facial steam to clear sinus infections.
- **Thyme** contains vitamin B6, vitamin C, vitamin A, lutein, potassium, iron, magnesium, and selenium. It's antispasmodic, antibacterial, and antimicrobial. It also aids digestion and brain function.
- **Turmeric** contains niacin, vitamin C, vitamin E, vitamin K, potassium, calcium, iron, magnesium, and zinc. It is a powerful immune booster and antioxidant. It fights arthritis and cancer, detoxifies the liver, and aids cognitive function.

A note about tomato sauce: Canned tomato sauce contains citric acid. This extra acidity makes tomato sauce especially problematic for people who have eczema, psoriasis, acid reflux, or arthritis, thus increasing its reactivity rate. Bottled tomato sauce usually does not contain citric acid, automatically making it less inflammatory. Tomato sauce can also be more reactive because of its sodium levels—most are so darn high in sodium! Sodium can really amplify a negative response, making a mildly inflammatory food wildly inflammatory. So take a look at the nutrition label and avoid the bottled tomato sauce with 600 milligrams of sodium and instead opt for the sauces that contain 300 milligrams or less.

Now, tomato sauce was pretty high on our devil food list, but I found a wonderful way to greatly decrease its reactivity, and it's all thanks to my little guy, Brayden. Anyone who has a picky kid knows what it's like to get them to eat foods they wouldn't normally eat. You know the drill, parents: Cook vegetables, puree them, and try to sneak them into other foods. I found that when I mixed Carrot Ginger Soup (page 101) with tomato sauce the taste was virtually unchanged. So in Brayden's case, I added in extra butternut squash and even beets—all was gobbled up as long as it was in Mama's secret sauce (aka Low-Reactive Tomato Sauce [page 137]). Did he flinch when he knew beets were in there? Yup! Did it stop him from eating it? Bless his little heart, it didn't! The great news? I was mildly reactive to tomato sauce, but found I could have it when I made it for Brayden. We have since used it with many of our Planners and have found that they can once again enjoy tomato sauce in moderation. So if you have given up this tasty little treat, give it a shot again with one of our recipes!

Melissa, 58

I'm in love with all of these new spices, like cardamom, turmeric, and cumin. Cooking so much of my food has given me a heightened sense of smell and taste. Everything I eat is delicious, brighter, and more fragrant!

Sauces

SPICY COCO SAUCE

Our classic sauce used for the cleanse and beyond. Planners like to make a big batch and freeze the sauce in ice cube trays for a quick, flavorful solution for vegetable sautées.

3 tbsp extra virgin olive oil

1 large onion, chopped fine

4 to 5 cloves garlic, minced

2-inch piece fresh ginger, peeled and grated (about 1 tbsp)

2 tsp ground cumin

1 tsp ground cinnamon

1 tsp freshly ground black pepper

1 tsp coriander

1 tsp nutmeg

1 tsp cardamom

½ tsp allspice

2 (14-oz) can full-fat unsweetened coconut milk

4 tbsp Sriracha, or more for extra spice

1 tsp brown sugar

Optional: 1 lemongrass stalk, cut into 1-inch pieces

In a large saucepan, heat olive oil over medium heat. Add onion and garlic and sauté until they start to brown. Add ginger, cumin, cinnamon, pepper, coriander, nutmeg, cardamom, and allspice and sauté for 1 minute at low heat, until spices start to smell fragrant. Add coconut milk, Sriracha, brown sugar, and lemongrass, if desired, stirring for 30 seconds. Reduce heat and simmer, stirring every 5 minutes, for 15 to 20 minutes, so flavors can fully integrate. Remove lemongrass. Serve immediately or let cool and then freeze.

Makes 4 to 6 servings (1½ cups)

SUNFLOWER BUTTER SATE

Sates are a wonderful way to brighten up the flavors of steamed, grilled, or sautéed vegetables, plus you get a nice protein boost!

¾ cup low-sodium or homemade chicken or vegetable stock

½ cup sunflower seed butter

Juice of 1 lime (1½ to 2 tbsp)

3 tbsp Sriracha

2 tsp ground ginger

3 garlic cloves, minced

1 Vietnamese chili pepper, minced, for garnish

¼ cup home-roasted sunflower seeds (see Roasted Nuts, page 115), for garnish

Combine stock, sunflower seed butter, lime juice, Sriracha, ginger, and garlic in food processor and blend well. Garnish sauce with chopped chili and roasted sunflower seeds. Refrigerate up to 1 week.

Makes 8 to 10 servings (1½ cups)

HARISSA

Harissa is a staple sauce in North Africa and the Middle East, and recipes range from mild to smoky or spicy and sweat inducing. The milder recipes often call for paprika, which can be reactive, while hotter chilies make this version more Plan friendly.

8 dried red chili peppers

2 cups hot water

1 tsp ground coriander

½ tsp caraway seeds

½ tsp ground cumin

½ tsp dried mint

4 tbsp extra virgin olive oil, plus more for serving

3 cloves garlic, minced

½ tsp sea salt

Soak dried chilies in hot water for 30 minutes. Drain. Halve chilies and remove stems and seeds.

Combine coriander, caraway, and cumin in a dry small skillet over medium heat and toast, shaking the pan, until fragrant. Transfer spices to a spice grinder or coffee grinder, add mint, and grind to a fine powder.

In a food processor, combine chilies, olive oil, garlic, and salt. Blend. Add ground spices and blend to form a smooth paste. Store in an airtight container. The sauce will keep for a month in the refrigerator. Drizzle a small amount of extra virgin olive oil on top when serving.

Makes 10 to 12 servings (¼ cup)

LOW-REACTIVE TOMATO SAUCE

1 (24-oz) bottle low-sodium tomato sauce

2½ cups Carrot Ginger Soup (page 101)

1 garlic clove, minced

2 tbsp dried basil

1 tbsp dried oregano

½ tsp dried rosemary

Optional: add 1 tbsp agave nectar or honey for pizza sauce.

Combine all ingredients in a large saucepan and simmer over low heat for 20 minutes. Let cool and pour into individual containers for freezing.

Makes 3 pints

ORANGE ZEST BUTTER

¼ cup (½ stick) unsalted butter, softened

2 tsp honey

1 tsp grated organic orange zest

In a small bowl, or with a hand mixer, cream butter with honey and orange zest until light and fluffy.

Makes 2 to 4 servings (¼ cup)

FIG VINEGAR

I love fig vinegar, but it can be really pricey! So take advantage of the bounty when figs are in season and make your own batch. Figs give an extra sweetness and depth to the balsamic vinegar, and it's great drizzled on a salad or meat. I also love reducing it to drizzle on berries, cheese, or duck.

    1 cup chopped fresh figs
    2 cups balsamic vinegar
    1 tbsp honey or agave nectar

Bring figs, vinegar, and honey or agave to a simmer in a medium saucepan over low heat. Cook, stirring occasionally, for 10 minutes, until figs are softened and tender. Cover and let cool completely. Transfer to the refrigerator and marinate for 24 hours.

Puree mixture in a food processor until smooth. Strain puree through a fine sieve into a large glass mixing cup. Pour into a cruet. The vinegar will keep for 2 weeks.

Makes 16 servings (1 pint)

GINGER DRESSING

    2 medium carrots, roughly chopped
    1 cup water
    3 tbsp chopped peeled fresh ginger
    1 tsp light brown sugar
    2 tbsp rice vinegar (natural, not seasoned)
    1 tsp fresh lemon juice
    ⅛ tsp sea salt
    Optional: 1 tsp sesame oil (see Note)

Bring carrots and water to a simmer in a small saucepan over medium-low heat. Cook until the carrots are tender, about 10 minutes.

Transfer carrots and ½ cup of the cooking liquid to a food processor. Add ginger, brown sugar, vinegar, lemon juice, salt, and sesame oil, if using, and pulse until smooth.

Note: Sesame oil can be reactive for some people, so you can use this recipe as a test to see if you can tolerate it. Make sure your sesame oil is not past its expiration date so there is lessened chance of rancidity.

Makes 4 to 6 servings (1 cup)

BERRY CHUTNEY

½ cup fresh or frozen blueberries

1 tbsp fresh lime juice (about ½ lime)

1 to 2 tbsp chipotle powder

1 tbsp agave nectar

½ tsp grated organic lime zest

Combine all ingredients except lime zest in a small saucepan and simmer for 5 minutes. Transfer to a food processor and puree. Pour chutney into a small jar and stir in lime zest. Serve or refrigerate for up to 1 week.

Makes 2 to 4 servings

CREAMY CUCUMBER SAUCE

2 cups chopped seeded cucumbers

6 oz goat cheese

¼ cup thinly sliced scallions

2 tsp chopped fresh mint

½ tsp ground cumin

⅛ tsp freshly ground black pepper

Combine all ingredients in a food processor. Pulse for 30 to 60 seconds for chunky sauce, 2 minutes for smooth. Store in refrigerator and use within 3 days.

Makes 6 to 8 servings (1½ cups)

PERSIAN POMEGRANATE SAUCE

Pomegranate sauce, used as a base for many Persian recipes, is chock-full of anti-oxidants. It's amazing on duck, chicken, and cake!

    3 cups pomegranate juice
    ⅓ cup sugar
    2 tbsp fresh lemon juice (½ to 1 lemon)
    1 tsp ground cinnamon
    1 tsp cardamom

Combine all ingredients in a saucepan and simmer over medium heat for 75 to 90 minutes, until reduced to ½ cup. Keep refrigerated in airtight container for up to 2 weeks.

Makes 4 to 6 servings (½ cup)

HEMP SEED PESTO

Hands down, this is a vegan Plan favorite for boosting protein at meals!

    2 cups packed fresh basil leaves
    ¾ cup hemp seeds
    ⅔ cup extra virgin olive oil
    2 cloves garlic, peeled
    1 tbsp balsamic vinegar

Combine all ingredients in a food processor and blend completely. Use immediately or freeze for up to 6 months.

Makes 6 servings (1 cup)

LEMON SUNFLOWER PESTO

    ¾ cup raw sunflower seeds
    1 cup water, plus more as needed

2 cups fresh basil leaves

½ cup fresh mint

1 cup extra virgin olive oil

1 tbsp balsamic vinegar, plus more as needed

2 cloves garlic, peeled

2 tbsp fresh lemon juice

Soak sunflower seeds in the water overnight. Drain.

Combine drained seeds and remaining ingredients in a food processor. Blend until smooth. To thin pesto, add water or more balsamic vinegar.

Note: You can substitute 2 cups fresh parsley or cilantro for the basil.

Makes 10 to 12 servings (1½ cups)

ADOBO SAUCE

Adobo is a sauce typically used in Mexican cooking and utilized as a marinade, during cooking, and as a delicious dipping sauce

8 dried ancho chili peppers

1 cup hot water

½ tsp dried oregano

1 tsp ground cumin

½ tsp ground cinnamon

⅛ tsp ground allspice

1 pinch ground cloves

¼ cup plus 2 tbsp minced onion

¼ cup minced garlic

2 tbsp fresh lime juice (about 1 lime)

1 tbsp brown sugar

½ tsp sea salt

Heat a dry large skillet over medium heat and toast the chilies, turning frequently, until soft. Transfer to a plate and let cool slightly. Halve chilies and remove stems and seeds. Combine chilies and hot water in a saucepan and bring to a simmer. Cover and simmer for 15 minutes. Drain through a fine mesh sieve over a bowl, reserving ¼ cup of cooking liquid.

In a dry small saucepan over medium heat, toast oregano, cumin, cinnamon, allspice, and cloves until fragrant.

Combine chilies, toasted spices, onion, garlic, lime juice, sugar, and salt in a food processor and puree. Add 2 to 4 tbsp of reserved chili liquid to make the sauce thinner, as desired.

Makes 16 to 20 servings (1½ cups)

SPICY BAHARAT RUB

Baharat is a Middle Eastern rub that is used on meats and vegetables; it is also very tasty when cooking grains like rice. We love it on The Plan because it's a flavorful, salt-free blend that is dynamite for digestion.

2 tbsp cayenne
1½ tsp ground cinnamon
1½ tsp ground coriander
1½ tsp ground cumin
1 tsp ground nutmeg
1 tsp dried thyme
½ tsp cardamom
⅛ tsp ground cloves
Optional: ¼ cup extra virgin olive oil

In a dry small saucepan over medium heat, toast all spices until fragrant. If desired, add toasted spices to olive oil. Store in an airtight container and use within 1 week for the freshest flavor.

Makes 4 servings (about ½ cup dry, ¾ cup with olive oil)

SWEET 'N' SOUR SAUCE

I love this as a quick easy sauce for duck; it's also a great spicy marinade for chicken wings.

¼ cup agave nectar

¼ cup rice vinegar (natural, not seasoned)

2 tbsp Sriracha

Combine ingredients in a cruet and shake until mixed. Serve or refrigerate for up to 5 days.

Makes 4 servings

AIOLI

I remember the first time I had a garlicky aioli with crudités, so simple, so heavenly. This is also a keeper for burgers, crab cakes, and sandwiches!

1 large egg yolk (see Note)

2 tsp water

3 small garlic cloves, finely grated

¼ tsp sea salt

½ cup extra virgin olive oil

Pinch of cayenne pepper

1 tsp lemon juice

½ tsp dried tarragon or herbs of choice

Freshly ground black pepper

In a small metal bowl, whisk egg yolk, water, garlic, and salt to blend well. Continue to whisk and drizzle in olive oil, 1 teaspoon at a time, until sauce is thickened and emulsified. Add cayenne, lemon juice, tarragon, and black pepper. Enjoy immediately.

Note: Raw egg is not recommended for infants, the elderly, pregnant women, and people with weakened immune systems.

Makes 6 to 8 servings (about ½ cup)

LEMON DILL SAUCE

Lemon and dill are a classic combination, delicious with fish, chicken, or vegetables.

¼ cup chopped fresh dill

2 cloves garlic, peeled

Grated zest and juice of 1 organic lemon

1½ tsp freshly ground black pepper

⅛ tsp sea salt

½ cup extra virgin olive oil

Combine dill, garlic, lemon zest and juice, pepper, and salt in a food processor and pulse until coarsely chopped. Continue pulsing while slowly drizzling in olive oil. Serve immediately.

Makes 4 to 6 servings

ORANGE THYME SAUCE

A perfect accompaniment to pork or lamb.

½ cup extra virgin olive oil

¼ cup balsamic vinegar

½ tsp grated organic orange zest

1 tsp dried basil

1 tsp dried thyme

1 tsp onion powder

Optional: 1 tsp agave nectar

Combine all ingredients in a cruet and shake. Serve immediately.

Makes 4 servings (¾ cup)

CRANBERRY CHUTNEY

A classic Thanksgiving side, chock-full of Vitamin C.

1 lb fresh or frozen cranberries

1 cup water

½ cup packed brown sugar

¼ cup chopped apple

2 tsp ground cinnamon

2 tsp grated peeled fresh ginger

½ tsp cardamom

½ tsp allspice

¼ cup almond slivers

½ tsp grated organic orange zest

Combine all ingredients except almond slivers and orange zest in a medium saucepan. Bring to a boil over medium heat, then reduce heat and simmer for about 10 minutes, until cranberries start to pop. Add almonds and orange zest and cook, stirring frequently, for 2 minutes, to break down cranberries for a chunky puree.

Makes 4 servings (2 cups)

SPICY APRICOT SAUCE

This sauce is so quick and easy you won't believe it. Many Planners who are new to cooking love using this sauce and impress people with their brand-new skills in the kitchen!

¾ cup apricot jam

¼ cup water

2 tbsp sriracha or 1 tbsp smoked chipotle powder

Combine all ingredients in a food processor and blend until smooth.

Makes 8 to 10 servings (1 cup)

ROSEMARY GARLIC SAUCE

The easiest way to make this sauce is to buy garlic that has already been peeled.

  20 large cloves garlic, peeled (or large cloves from 4 heads of garlic)

  ¾ cup extra virgin olive oil

  2 tbsp lemon juice

  2 tbsp balsamic vinegar

  2 tbsp rosemary

Preheat oven to 275°F. Place garlic on an ungreased baking sheet and roast for 30 minutes, until slightly tender and lightly browned. Let cool for 5 minutes. Combine roasted garlic with remaining ingredients in a food processor and blend until smooth, 1 to 2 minutes. Store in an airtight container and use within 5 days or freeze.

Makes 8 to 10 servings (1½ cups)

QUICK AND EASY PICKLED GINGER

I love pickled ginger with sashimi but it often has dye, MSG, and way too much sodium. Try this fast, delicious, and digestive-boosting recipe for a healthier option!

  3 inches peeled fresh ginger

  ½ cup Sweet 'n' Sour Sauce (page 143)

  2 tbsp rice vinegar (natural, not seasoned)

  1 tbsp Sriracha

Slice ginger into very thin rounds about ¹⁄₁₆ inch thick. Combine sweet and sour sauce, rice vinegar, and Sriracha in a small glass jar. Place ginger in jar and let marinate for at least 4 hours. Ginger is good refrigerated for up to 1 week.

Makes 2 to 4 servings

APPLE BOURBON SAUCE

You can use any dark alcohol, but bourbon has this lovely vanilla taste that pairs so well with apples! Serve immediately so the flavors don't dissipate. I have served this on venison, duck, and even ice cream.

- 2 tbsp unsalted butter
- 1 tsp ground cinnamon
- ¼ tsp ground cloves
- ½ tsp freshly ground black pepper
- 2 medium apples, peeled, cored, and diced
- ½ cup bourbon

Melt butter in a small skillet over medium heat. Add spices and sauté for 20 seconds. Add apples and stir for 15 seconds, until apples are coated with spices. Add bourbon and simmer for 10 to 12 minutes, until apples are completely softened. Remove from heat and serve immediately for best flavor.

Makes 4 to 6 servings (2 cups)

MANGO SALSA

Many fruits will work for salsa; mango is a great low-reactive start.

- 1 mango, pitted, peeled, and chopped; or 1 cup thawed frozen mango
- ½ small red onion, chopped (¼ cup)
- Juice of 1 lime (1½ to 2 tbsp)
- 1 small dried red chili pepper, cut into strips
- 1 tbsp grated peeled fresh ginger

Combine all ingredients in a small mixing bowl. Serve immediately or refrigerate for up to 5 days.

Makes 4 to 6 servings (1¼ cups)

QUICK AND EASY RANCHERO SAUCE

Tomato sauce can be reactive, but when mixed with Carrot Ginger Soup (page 101) it becomes *much* more friendly. This is changing the dietary landscape for so many Planners!

½ tsp ground cumin

½ tsp chipotle powder

1 tbsp extra virgin olive oil

2 cloves garlic, chopped

¼ cup Low-Reactive Tomato Sauce (page 137)

¼ cup Carrot Ginger Soup (page 101)

¼ cup chopped red onion

Juice of 1 lime (1½ to 2 tbsp)

Dash of agave nectar

In a small dry skillet, toast cumin and chipotle over medium heat until fragrant. Add oil and garlic and sauté for 1 minute, until garlic starts to brown. Add tomato sauce and soup and cook, stirring, for 1 minute. Transfer to a bowl and mix in red onion, lime juice, and agave. Serve immediately or refrigerate for up to 5 days

Makes 4 servings (½ cup)

Salad Dressings

LIME AGAVE VINAIGRETTE

This is our standard dressing for the cleanse and replaces vinegar when fighting yeast. Of course you can always use fresh lemon juice, olive oil, and the herbs of your choice!

¼ cup freshly squeezed lime juice (2 to 3 limes)

¼ cup extra virgin olive oil

2 tbsp water

1 tbsp agave nectar

1 clove garlic, crushed

Optional: 1 tsp dried dill

Combine all ingredients in a cruet and mix thoroughly. Toss with any salad of your choosing. Will keep refrigerated in an airtight container for up to 1 week.

Makes 6 servings (¾ cup)

PLAN CAESAR DRESSING

This delicious dressing adds extra protein to your salads, making them a healthy weight loss wonder.

2 cloves garlic, chopped

¼ cup extra virgin olive oil

4 oz goat cheese

2 tbsp lemon juice

2 tsp fresh black pepper

Optional: 2 tbsp chopped fresh dill or basil

Soak chopped garlic in olive oil overnight. Transfer to a food processor, add remaining ingredients, and blend until smooth. Add water as needed for lighter dressing. Store in fridge for up to 5 days.

Makes 4 servings (about ½ cup)

DAIRY-FREE CAESAR DRESSING

Remember when you see hemp, think "protein rich." Hemp is delicious and reminds me of a mix of cheese, couscous, and pine nuts.

2 cloves garlic, chopped

¼ cup extra virgin olive oil

¼ cup hemp seeds

2 tbsp lemon juice

2 tsp freshly ground black pepper

Optional: 2 tbsp fresh dill or basil

Soak chopped garlic cloves in olive oil overnight. Transfer to a food processor, add remaining ingredients, and blend until smooth. Add water as needed for lighter dressing.

Makes 4 servings (about ½ cup)

OREGANO GARLIC VINAIGRETTE

For many people with yeast conditions, balsamic vinegar is not encouraged because it can promote yeast growth. This can be tough, because it really does make such a fantastic salad dressing. The solution may be to use this vinaigrette recipe because garlic, oregano, and rosemary all do a great job at fighting yeast!

½ cup extra virgin olive oil

¼ cup balsamic vinegar

2 cloves garlic, crushed

1 tsp dried rosemary

1 tsp dried oregano

Mix all ingredients together in a cruet and let marinate for a minimum of 2 hours. Use within 4 days.

Makes 6 servings (about ¾ cup)

DAIRY-FREE RANCH DRESSING

1 cup canned full-fat unsweetened coconut milk

2 tbsp fresh lemon juice

1 tsp balsamic vinegar

¼ cup Aioli (page 143) or store-bought mayo

2 tbsp finely minced chives

1 tsp honey or agave nectar

1 tsp garlic powder

1 tsp onion powder

½ tsp freshly ground black pepper

½ tsp dried sage

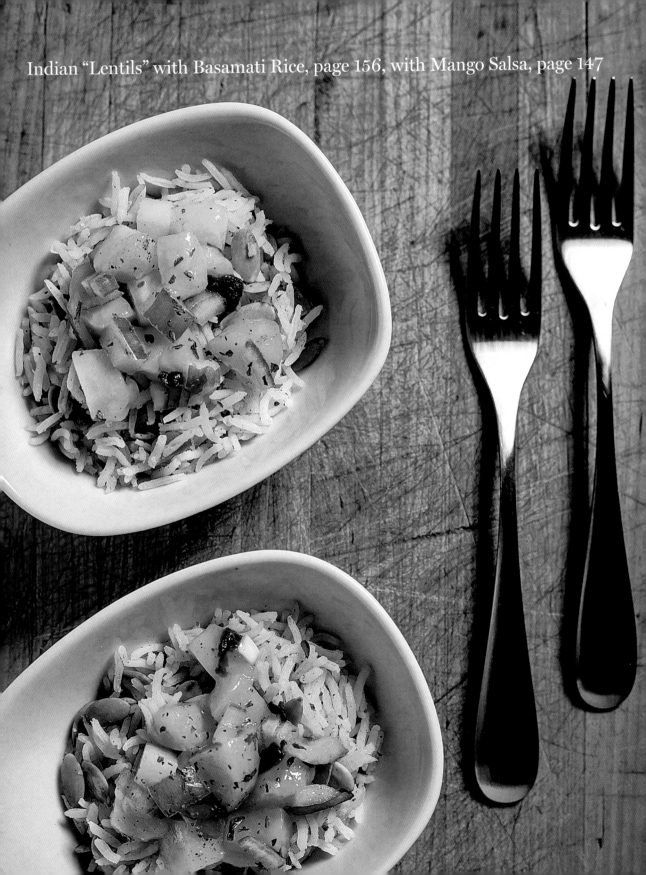

Indian "Lentils" with Basamati Rice, page 156, with Mango Salsa, page 147

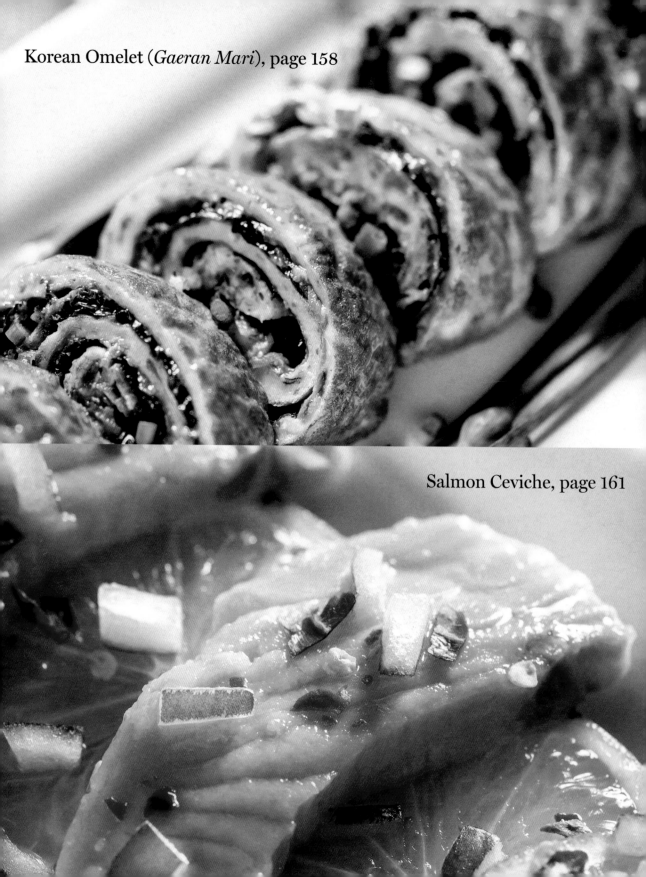

Korean Omelet (*Gaeran Mari*), page 158

Salmon Ceviche, page 161

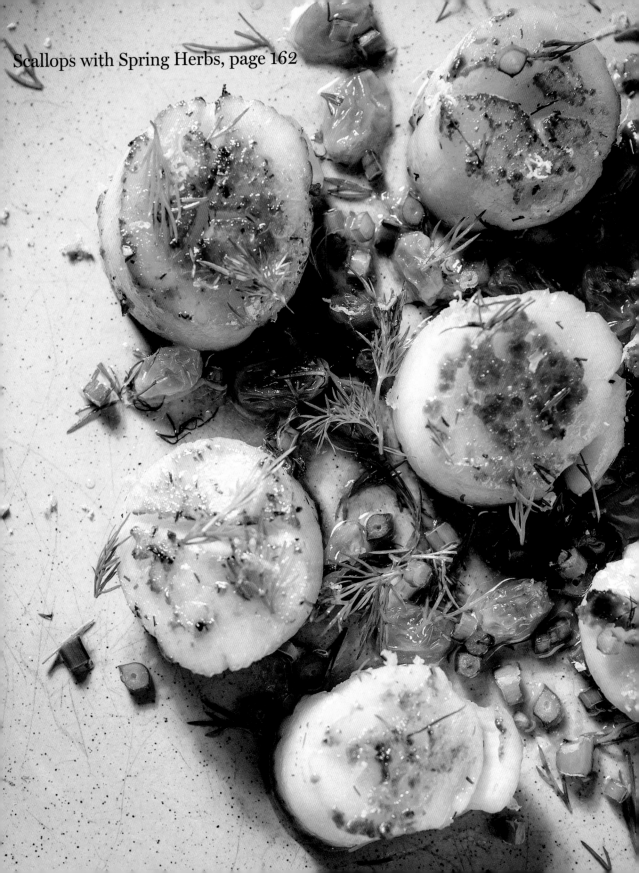

Scallops with Spring Herbs, page 162

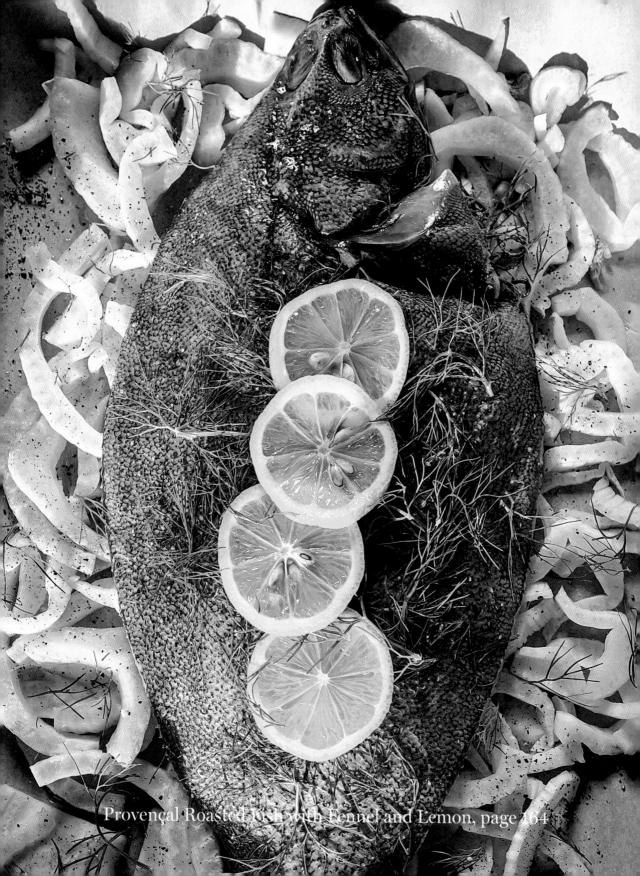

Provençal Roasted Fish with Fennel and Lemon, page 164

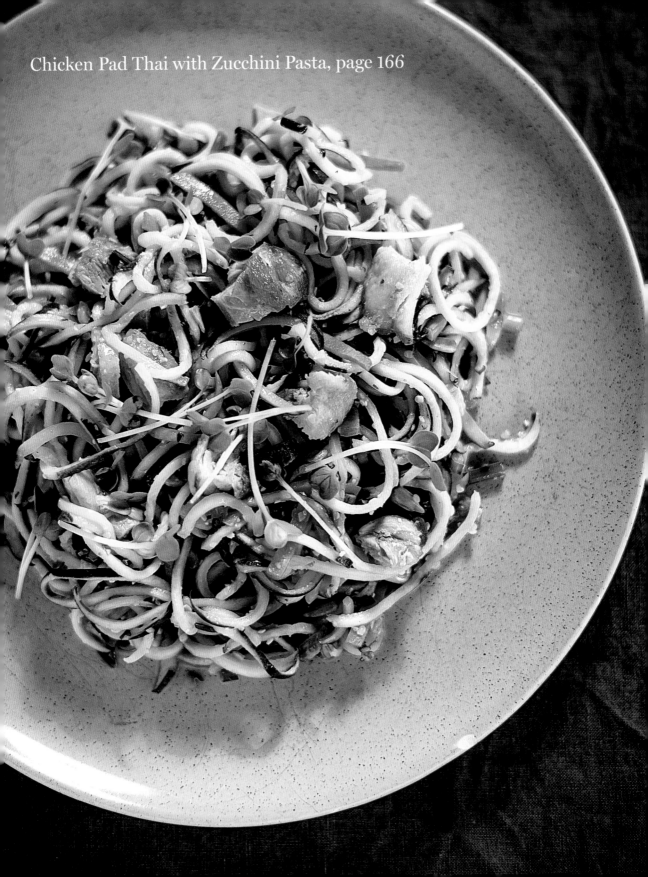

Chicken Pad Thai with Zucchini Pasta, page 166

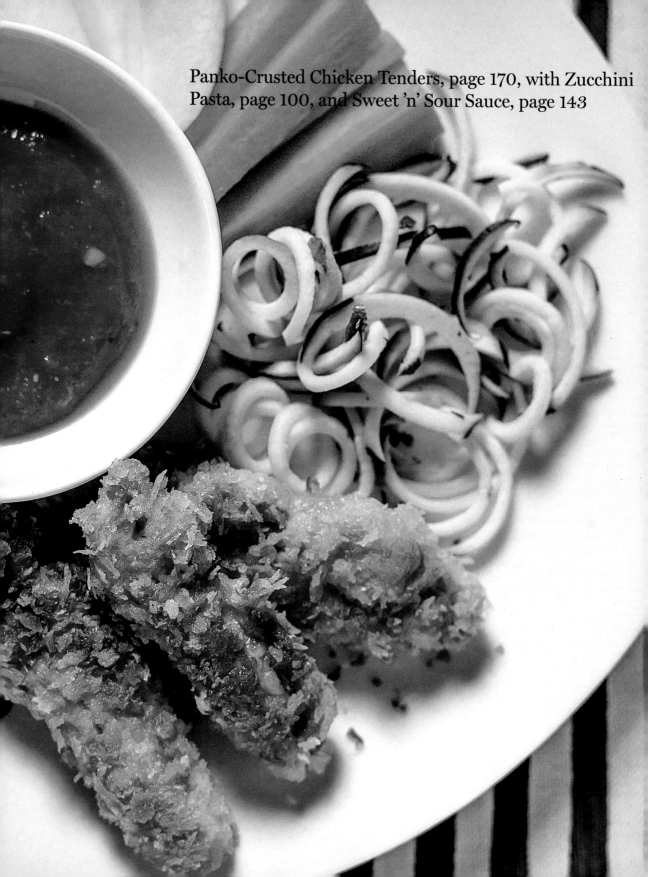

Panko-Crusted Chicken Tenders, page 170, with Zucchini Pasta, page 100, and Sweet 'n' Sour Sauce, page 143

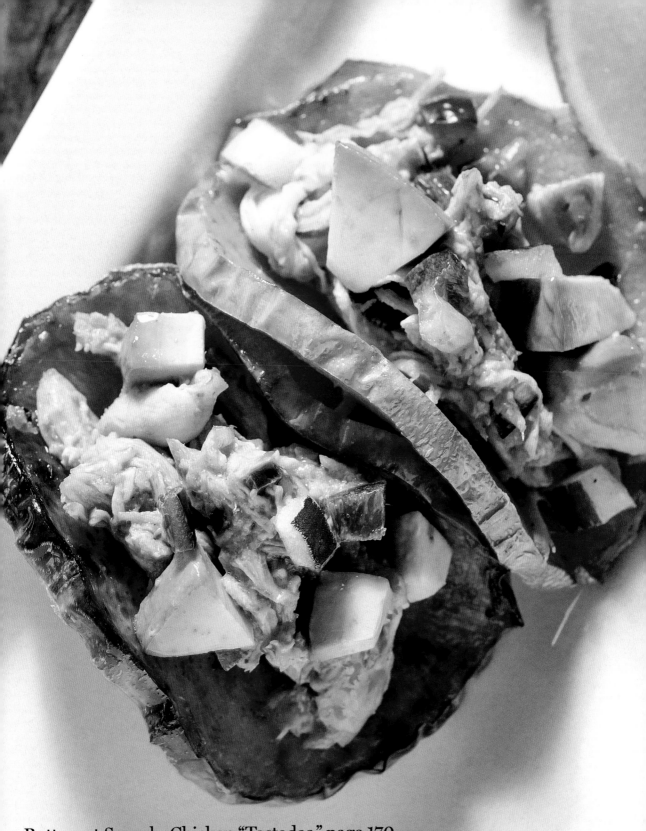

Butternut Squash–Chicken "Tostadas," page 170

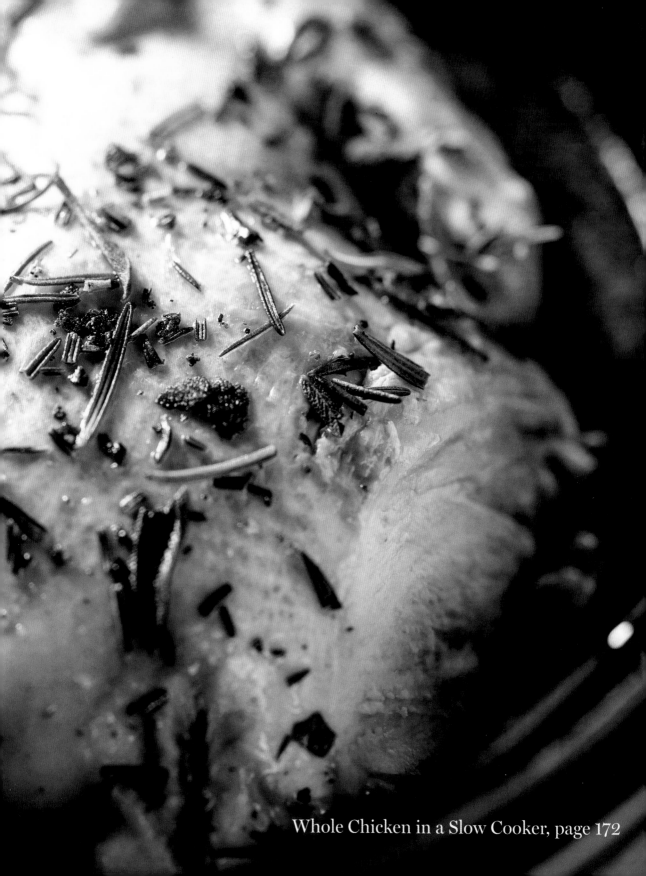

Whole Chicken in a Slow Cooker, page 172

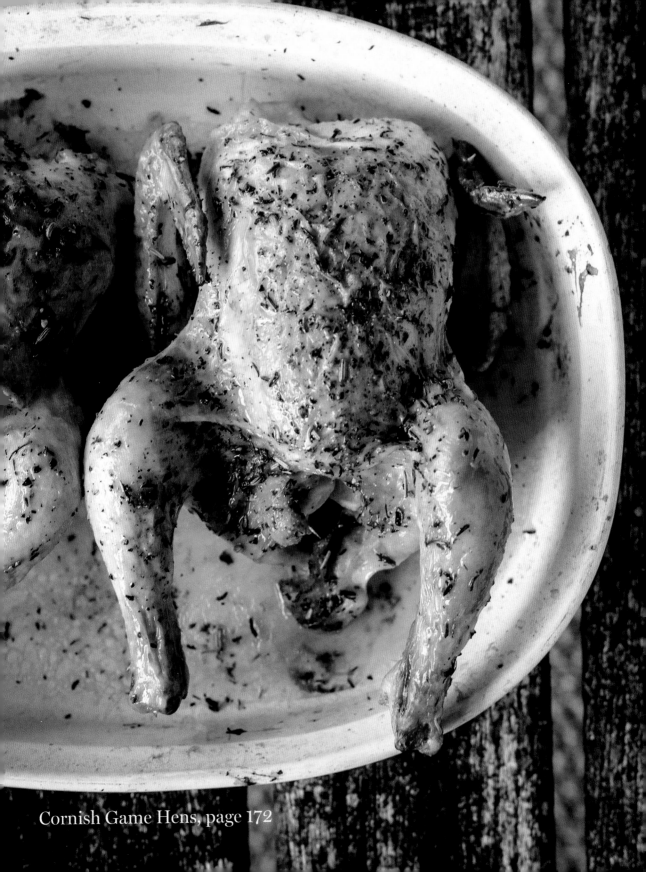

Cornish Game Hens, page 172

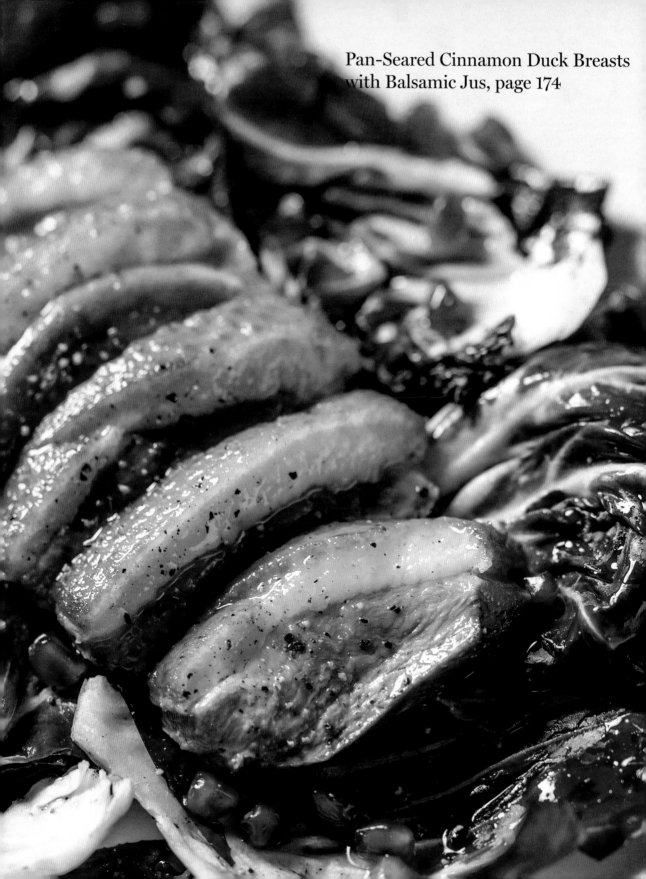

Pan-Seared Cinnamon Duck Breasts
with Balsamic Jus, page 174

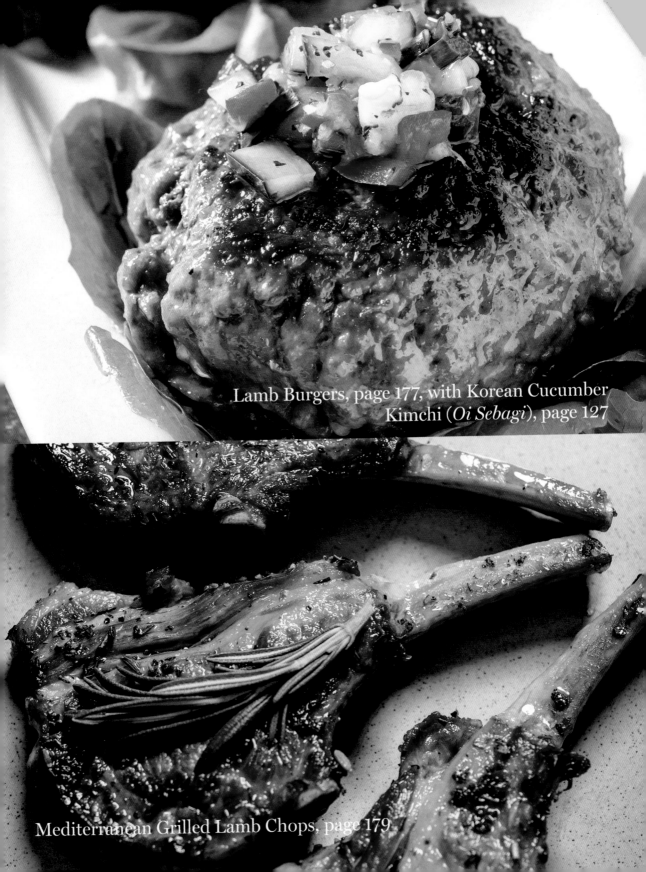

Lamb Burgers, page 177, with Korean Cucumber Kimchi (*Oi Sebagi*), page 127

Mediterranean Grilled Lamb Chops, page 179

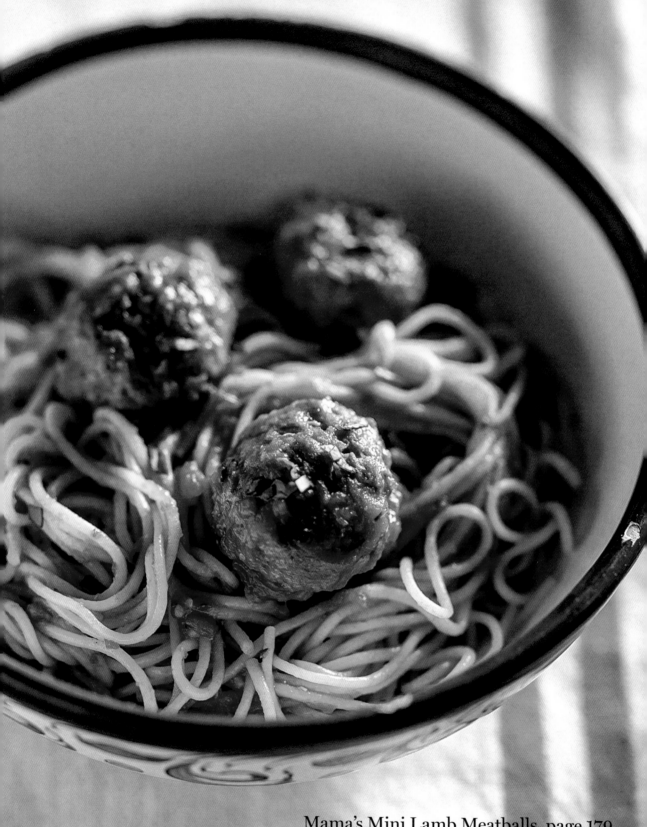

Mama's Mini Lamb Meatballs, page 179

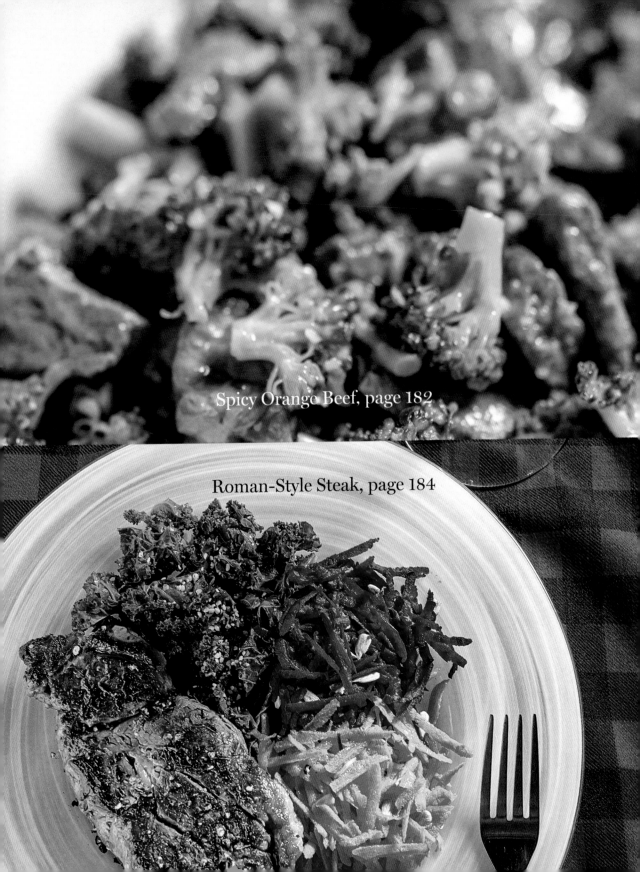

Spicy Orange Beef, page 182

Roman-Style Steak, page 184

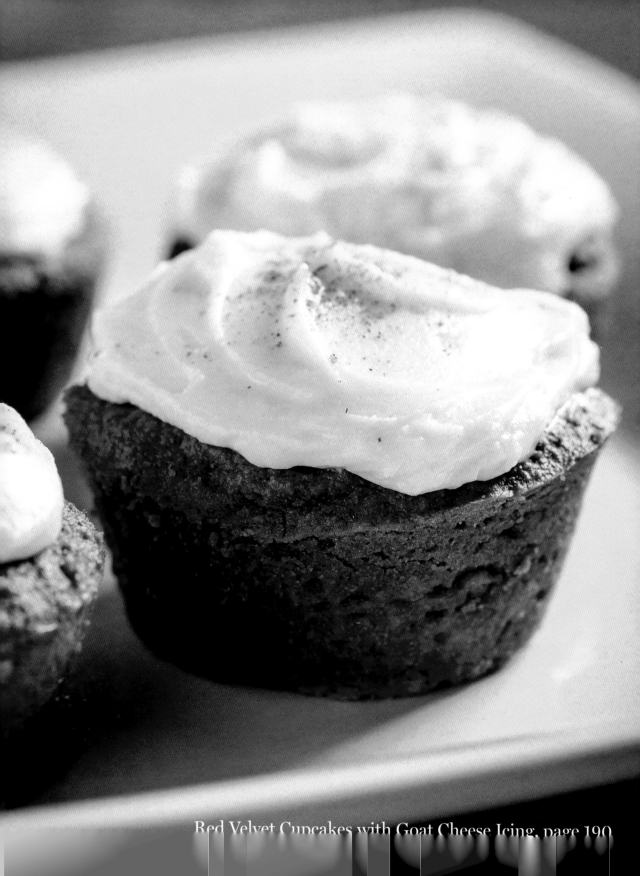

Red Velvet Cupcakes with Goat Cheese Icing, page 190

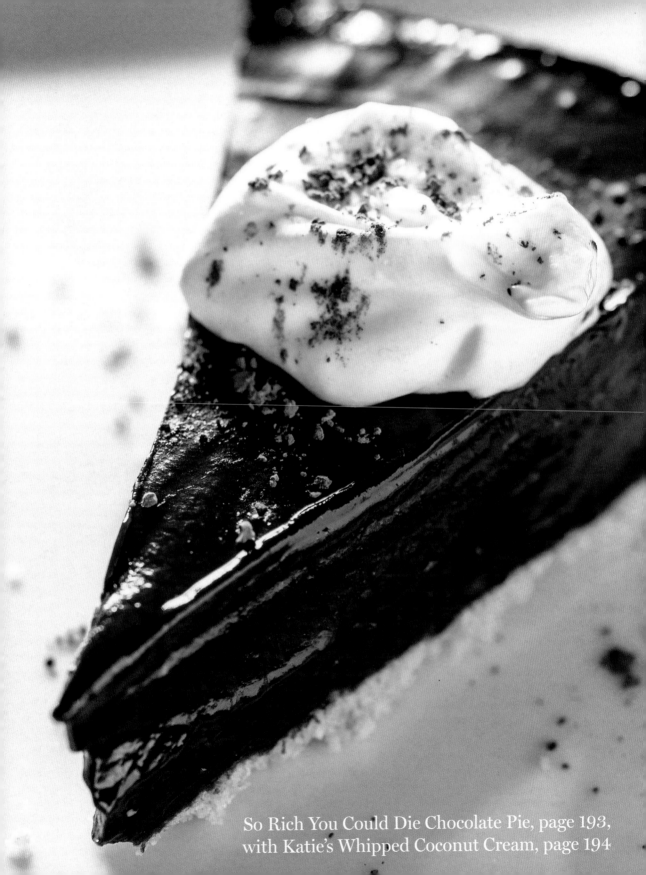

So Rich You Could Die Chocolate Pie, page 193,
with Katie's Whipped Coconut Cream, page 194

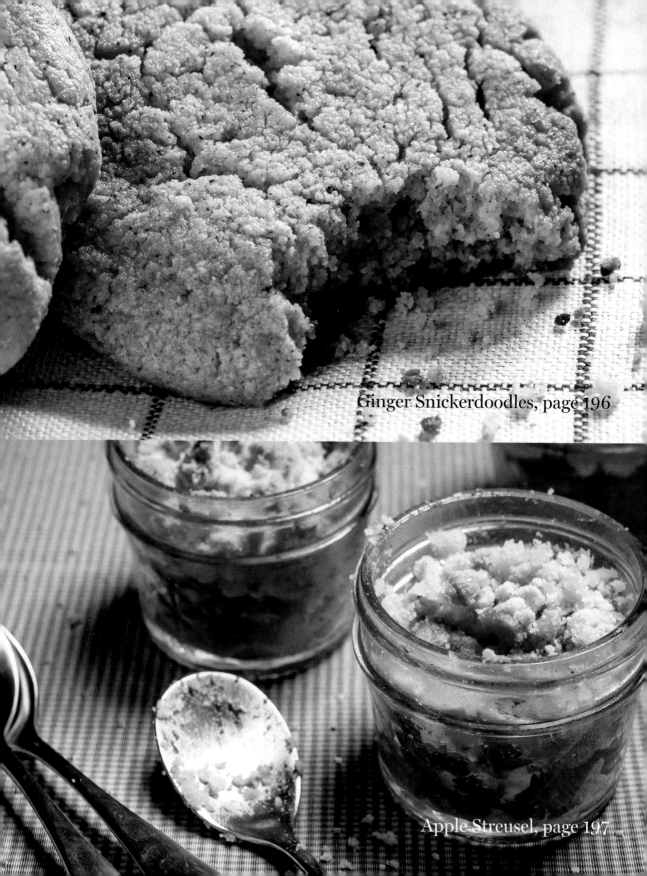

Ginger Snickerdoodles, page 196

Apple Streusel, page 197

In a small bowl, whisk coconut milk with lemon juice and vinegar; let sit for 5 minutes. Whisk in remaining ingredients until dressing is smooth and creamy. Cover and refrigerate for at least 30 minutes to allow the flavors to meld and the dressing to thicken.

Makes 10 to 12 servings (about 1½ cups)

CHIPOTLE-AVO DRESSING

A smoky dressing to beef up grilled vegetables. In the mood for something mild? Just leave out the chipotle and enjoy the creaminess.

    2 medium avocados, peeled and pitted
    3 tbsp lime juice
    ¼ cup extra virgin olive oil
    2 tbsp water
    1 tsp chipotle powder
    1 to 2 medium cloves garlic, crushed
    ¼ tsp sea salt

Combine all ingredients in a food processor and blend until smooth.

Makes 8 to 10 servings (about 2 cups)

LEMON POPPYSEED DRESSING

Sweet and sour with a delightful crunch. This dressing is great for salads or slaws.

    ⅔ cup extra virgin olive oil
    2 tbsp agave nectar
    2 tbsp lemon juice
    2 tbsp poppyseeds
    1 tbsp balsamic vinegar
    ½ tsp grated organic lemon zest

Combine all ingredients in a cruet and shake to mix. Serve immediately or store in the fridge for up to 2 days.

Makes 8 servings (about 1 cup)

Entrees

Ahhhh, dinner. My favorite meal of the day. A time to relax and enjoy.

My days are a whirlwind of activity (probably like yours), and I'm going nonstop for most of it. In fact, I'm a nutritionist's nightmare! I eat too fast, I eat standing up. Sometimes I forget to eat because my day is so stressful and next thing you know I am starving, eating cheese and crackers with Sriracha like some sort of inhaling machine.

But dinner is the beginning of happy time. I get to unwind, listen to my favorite music, have a glass of wine, and create dishes for my family and friends. It's always my biggest meal of the day, and I love making two or three quick side dishes and a main course. My way of showing my love for family and friends is through the kitchen—I cook. It's the one thing I will always have for you if you come to my house. Lots of food.

Because I'm so busy and work up until seconds before I start dinner, I have always been the queen of the quick cook. Would I like to have time to dance around and massage a chicken under a full moon, gathering the herbs from my garden to season it? You bet, but my lifestyle's not that way and I have a feeling yours isn't either. Perhaps it will be when I retire, but for now I want to eat and serve delicious food that's quick and easy to prepare.

The recipes in this chapter are the simplest ways I can make food that my family and friends love. Share them with the people close to you—they will feel nourished and happy. In fact, I hope you have at least four big belly laughs with each dinner. These recipes are my hug to you, dear friend—so break out a glass of wine, sharpen those knives, and let's get cooking!

INDIAN "LENTILS" WITH BASMATI RICE

The combo of beans and rice can become much more inflammatory as we age, but the good news is that rice and seeds don't! The pumpkin seeds will stand in as a "bean" and the soaking process will make them more digestible, allowing greater absorption of the nutrients.

½ cup pumpkin seeds

3 cups water

1 tbsp extra virgin olive oil

1 tsp ground cumin

1 tsp ground cinnamon

½ tsp nutmeg

½ tsp cardamom

¼ tsp allspice

1 cup uncooked basmati rice

Optional: 1 to 2 tbsp unsalted butter, softened, or ghee

Optional: 2 tbsp raisins

Soak pumpkin seeds overnight in 1 cup water.

Rinse and drain pumpkin seeds. Heat olive oil in a saucepan over medium heat. Add cumin, cinnamon, nutmeg, cardamom, and allspice and sauté for 1 minute. Add pumpkin seeds and stir thoroughly.

Pour remaining 2 cups water into a saucepan, place over high heat, and bring to a boil. Add rice, cover, and reduce heat to low. Simmer for 20 to 22 minutes, until rice is completely cooked. Stir in butter or ghee and raisins, if desired. Combine with pumpkin seeds and serve.

Makes 4 servings

KALE IN SPICY COCO SAUCE

The cleanse classic!

2 tbsp extra virgin olive oil

1 large red onion, chopped

4 to 5 large cloves garlic, minced

1 tbsp grated peeled fresh ginger

1 tsp freshly ground black pepper

1 tsp ground cumin

½ tsp turmeric

½ tsp coriander

1 head kale, deveined and chopped (5 to 6 cups)

2 large zucchini, chopped

2 heads broccoli, chopped

1 lb carrots, chopped

4 shiitake mushrooms, diced

1 cup Carrot Soup Essence (page 102)

Spicy Coco Sauce (page 135)

Heat olive oil in an 8-quart soup pot over medium heat. Add onion, garlic, ginger, pepper, cumin, turmeric, and coriander and sauté for 1 minute. Add kale, zucchini, broccoli, carrots, and mushrooms and stir so spice and onion mix is well integrated, 1 to 2 minutes. Add soup essence, cover, and reduce heat to lowest setting. Simmer for 20 minutes. Add spicy coco sauce and simmer for an additional 10 minutes, stirring frequently to integrate flavors.

Makes 4 servings

Roasted Jalapeño Peppers

8 to 10 jalapeños
Oil for baking sheet

Set oven to broil-high. Place jalapeños on oiled baking sheet and broil for 10 to 12 minutes, until skins are blackened. Flip jalapeños and broil on other side until skins are charred. Using gloves, remove peppers and place in a paper bag for 5 minutes, until the skins are loosened. Remove the peppers and use a spoon to scrape off the charred skin. Discard skin. Peppers will last for 1 to 2 weeks.

KOREAN OMELET (*GAERAN MARI*)

This is an incredibly elegant dish, and beautiful for brunch.

6 large eggs

½ tsp freshly ground black pepper

½ cup finely chopped red onion

¼ cup chopped baby kale

1 carrot, finely chopped or grated

1 tbsp extra virgin olive oil

1 sheet Maine Coast Sea Vegetables Sushi Nori

Optional garnish: 3 or 4 whole flower chives

Whisk eggs and pepper together for 1 minute. Stir in onion, kale, and carrot. Heat oil in a large sauté pan. Pour egg mixture into pan, and heat slowly over low heat for 2 to 3 minutes. Raise heat to medium and cook for 4 to 5 minutes longer, until you can lift browned egg with a spatula and top of omelet is firm and not runny. Flip omelet and cook for 1 to 2 additional minutes so both sides are browned. Remove omelet from pan.

To assemble, place seaweed on top of omelet. Roll omelet into a tight roll by lifting one side with a spatula. Let omelet rest for a few minutes to cool. Slice into 1-inch pieces and serve. Garnish with flower chives, if desired.

Makes 2 servings

TARRAGON AND GOAT RICOTTA FRITTATA

2 tbsp extra virgin olive oil

2 shallots, finely chopped

2 tsp dried tarragon

½ cup chopped deveined kale

⅛ tsp sea salt

¼ tsp freshly ground black pepper

Dash of rice cooking wine

8 large eggs

4 oz goat-cheese ricotta

Preheat oven to broil. Grease a cast-iron skillet with 1 tbsp olive oil and warm over medium heat. Add shallots and tarragon and cook, stirring, for 30 seconds. Add kale, salt, pepper, and rice wine and sauté for 2 to 3 minutes, until kale starts to wilt.

Beat eggs in a large mixing bowl for 1 minute, add ricotta, and mix until thoroughly combined. Add eggs to kale and sauté over medium heat for 2 to 3 minutes, until underside sets.

Transfer pan to oven, and broil for 4 to 5 minutes, until nicely browned. Let frittata cool for 2 to 3 minutes, then slice into quarters.

Makes 4 servings

CRUSTLESS LEEK AND SHIITAKE QUICHE

Of course you can make this with a crust; either way, this quick and easy dinner can't be beat.

Extra virgin olive oil spray (from an olive oil mister)

1 lb leeks

1 tbsp olive oil

½ cup shiitake mushrooms

6 large eggs

1 cup grated goat-cheese Gouda

1½ cups canned full-fat unsweetened coconut milk

1 tsp dried tarragon

½ tsp coarsely ground black pepper

Preheat oven to 350°F. Spray a pie plate with olive oil.

Cut off stems and dark green tops from leeks. Cut each leek in half, then into ¼-inch slices. Rinse leeks in a colander under cold water. Repeat until all sand is removed. Drain and pat dry with a paper or cloth napkin. Heat olive oil in a skillet over medium-low heat. Add leeks and cook for 6 minutes, then add shiitakes. Cook an additional 6 minutes.

Add leek-shiitake mixture to prepared pie plate. Whisk eggs, cheese, coconut milk, tarragon, and pepper together. Pour egg mixture over leeks. Bake quiche 30 to 35 minutes, until knife inserted in center comes out clean. Cool on a wire rack for 5 to 10 minutes. Cut into slices and serve warm or at room temperature.

Makes 4 to 6 servings

CHANA MASALA

Stewing chickpeas for a long time helps to break down cellulose, and the digestive spices of this version of chana masala have made the chickpeas even friendlier than usual!

2 tbsp extra virgin olive oil

1 tbsp ground cumin

1 tsp black pepper

1 tsp coriander

1 tsp ground cinnamon

½ tsp cardamom

1 large onion, chopped

4 cloves garlic, minced

2 tbsp peeled, grated fresh ginger (from 2-inch piece)

1 cup low-sodium or homemade chicken stock

½ cup water

¼ cup Low-Reactive Tomato Sauce (page 137)

2 cups chickpeas, drained and rinsed

4 cups chopped deveined kale

2 carrots, chopped

1 large zucchini, chopped

In a medium saucepan, heat olive oil over medium heat. Add spices and sauté for 2 minutes, until fragrant. Add onion, garlic, and ginger and cook 3 to 4 minutes, until onion starts to soften. Add all remaining ingredients and mix well. Cover and simmer, stirring occasionally, for 30 minutes, until the chickpeas are very tender. Serve warm.

Makes 4 servings

PLAN PIZZA

Lavash—an Armenian flatbread that you can get in many Middle Eastern stores—is a great choice for making Plan-friendly pizza, as it often contains no yeast or starter! If you can't find lavash, you can always use pita bread.

Extra virgin olive oil, for brushing

9x12-inch lavash

¼ cup Low-Reactive Tomato Sauce (page 137)

⅓ cup grated goat-cheese Cheddar

Optional toppings: chopped fresh basil, rosemary, or oregano

Preheat broiler. Brush a pizza pan or baking pan with olive oil and place lavash on pan. Spread tomato sauce on lavash and top with Cheddar. Place under broiler for 4 minutes, until cheese is browned. Top with fresh herbs if you like. Cut into slices and serve warm.

Makes 2 to 4 servings

SALMON CEVICHE

Some seasoned Planners may be wondering why I'm featuring a salmon recipe in the book, considering that salmon is one of the most highly reactive foods. Well, it's only *cooked* salmon that's the devil, my friend. Salmon sashimi, carpaccio, and ceviche range from 15 to 20 percent. So enjoy!

1 lb fresh wild salmon

3 tbsp extra virgin olive oil

Juice of 6 limes; plus 1 lime, sliced, for garnish

1 tsp honey

2 tbsp grated peeled fresh ginger

1 red chili pepper, finely chopped

¼ tsp salt

Optional: ¼ cup chopped cilantro

Optional: ¼ cup diced red onion

Pat salmon dry and slice into ¼-inch-thick slices. Whisk together oil, lime juice, honey, ginger, chili, and salt in a large bowl. Place salmon slices gently in bowl and let each piece soak in lime mixture for 5 to 10 minutes. Turn slices and let salmon soak completely on other side for 5 to 10 minutes.

Transfer salmon to a platter and garnish with cilantro and red onion, if desired, and sliced lime rounds.

Makes 4 servings

SCALLOPS WITH SPRING HERBS

1 tbsp extra virgin olive oil

1 lb large sea scallops

¼ tsp freshly ground black pepper

2 tbsp unsalted butter, cut into small pieces

¼ cup organic golden raisins

2 tbsp chopped fresh chives

2 tbsp chopped fresh tarragon

Lemon Dill Sauce (page 144) or Orange Thyme Sauce (page 144)

Heat olive oil in a large skillet over medium-high heat. Season scallops with pepper. Add scallops to skillet and cook until deep golden brown on one side, about 3 minutes. Turn scallops and add butter, raisins, and herbs to pan. Continue cooking, spooning butter over scallops often, until scallops are cooked through and butter is brown and smells nutty, about 3 minutes longer. Serve with sauce of choice.

Makes 4 servings

HALIBUT WITH JASMINE TEA BROTH

4 tbsp extra virgin olive oil

1 to 1½ lb halibut fillet, cut into 4 portions

1 tsp freshly ground black pepper

1 small white onion, finely chopped

2-inch piece fresh ginger, peeled and grated (about 1 tbsp)

4 shiitake mushrooms, chopped

1 clove garlic, chopped

2 cups Carrot Soup Essence (page 102)

3 cups chopped endive

1 cup julienned carrots

2 tbsp loose jasmine tea leaves

Preheat oven to 400°F. Oil a medium baking dish with 2 tbsp olive oil.

Season halibut with pepper. In a large skillet, heat 1 tbsp olive oil over medium-high heat. Add halibut and cook until slightly browned on each side, 2 to 3 minutes. Transfer fish to prepared baking dish and bake for 7 to 8 minutes, until cooked through.

Meanwhile, add remaining 1 tbsp olive oil to same large skillet and add onion, ginger, shiitakes, and garlic. Sauté for 1 minute. Add soup essence, endive, carrots, and tea leaves and simmer for 3 to 4 minutes, or until endive is wilted.

Spoon broth and vegetables over cooked fish before serving.

Makes 4 servings

GINGER-STEAMED WHOLE FISH

1 whole red snapper (1 to 2 lb), cleaned and scaled

½ tsp sea salt, plus additional pinch to make ginger paste

3-inch piece fresh ginger, peeled and grated (about 3 tbsp)

2 tsp sesame oil

8 scallions, finely julienned and then cut into 1-inch lengths

1 lemongrass stalk, cut into 1-inch diagonal pieces

4 cups water

1 tbsp extra virgin olive oil

2 tbsp rice vinegar (natural, not seasoned)

Wash fish in cold water and wipe dry. Place fish on a heat-proof plate and make 3 parallel diagonal 2-inch-long slits on each side of fish, slicing through to bone. Rub fish all over with ½ tsp salt.

In a mortar, pound ginger and 1 tsp sesame oil to a paste with a pinch of salt. Fill slits on both sides of fish with ginger-sesame paste. Tuck ¼ of scallion shreds and all of lemongrass into cavity of fish. Spoon any ginger from plate over fish.

Pour 4 cups water into a large wok and place a bamboo steamer above it. Set plate with fish in steamer and bring water to a boil. Do not let water touch steamer. Cover tightly with a lid. Steam fish until it is opaque throughout and flakes easily when pulled with a fork, 15 to 18 minutes.

Meanwhile, combine olive oil, remaining 1 tsp sesame oil, and remaining scallions in a cast-iron skillet and sauté for 30 seconds. Add rice vinegar and cook for 30 seconds.

Using oven mitts, carefully remove steamer from wok. Pour the hot oil mixture over fish to glaze it (steaming often leaves a very matte finish). Serve fish immediately from plate.

Makes 2 to 4 servings

PROVENÇAL ROASTED FISH WITH FENNEL AND LEMON

Celery is very reactive for most people, but it can be low reactive for those who have heart disease or blood pressure issues. Customize this recipe accordingly and leave out the celery if it doesn't work for you.

1 fennel bulb, trimmed (reserve stems and fronds), cored, sliced ⅛ to ¼ inch thick, and cut into thin strips

4 tbsp extra virgin olive oil

1 whole flounder (about 2½ lb)

½ tsp sea salt

1 tsp freshly ground black pepper

Optional: ¼ cup chopped celery

2 lemons, cut into very thin slices

¼ cup white wine

Preheat oven to 400°F.

Slice the stems and fronds off fennel bulb. Slice fennel into thin strips and reserve fronds and stems for fish cavity. Coat the bottom of a large roasting pan with parchment paper and 2 tbsp olive oil. Arrange fennel strips in an even layer to cover bottom. Rub fish inside and out with 1 tbsp olive oil and season with salt and pepper. Tuck some fennel fronds and stems in fish cavity, along with celery, if desired. Center fish on top of fennel. Cover fish with remaining fennel stems and fronds and the lemon slices. Drizzle fennel and fish with remaining 1 tbsp olive oil. Pour wine around fish.

Roast 30 to 35 minutes. You can test fish by inserting a fork: When it has no resistance, the fish is done. Let rest for 10 minutes and serve.

Note: The thinner you slice the fennel, the sweeter the flavor.

Makes 4 to 6 servings

CHICKEN WITH FENNEL-APPLE SALAD

¼ cup extra virgin olive oil

2 skinless boneless chicken breasts, chopped

1 large fennel bulb, trimmed and thinly sliced

¼ cup low-sodium or homemade chicken stock

2 medium apples, cored and sliced

¼ cup slivered almonds

½ cup Plan Guacamole (page 114)

Sea salt and freshly ground black pepper, to taste

1 tbsp organic dried cranberries

Heat olive oil in a large skillet over medium-high heat. Add chicken and fennel and sauté 5 minutes, until fennel is tender. Add stock and cook for 15 to 20 minutes, until chicken is cooked though. Let cool in fridge for at least 30 minutes or up to 24 hours.

Place chicken mixture, apples, and almonds in a salad bowl. Add guacamole and toss. Taste and season with salt and pepper. Top salad with cranberries and serve.

Option: Do not refrigerate and serve as a warm salad.

Makes 4 to 6 servings

CHICKEN PAD THAI WITH ZUCCHINI PASTA

4 tbsp extra virgin olive oil

3 tbsp rice vinegar (natural, not seasoned)

2 tbsp fresh lime juice

1 tbsp brown sugar

¼ tsp fish sauce

2 tbsp thinly sliced scallions

4 garlic cloves, finely minced (about 2 tbsp)

1 lb skinless boneless chicken breasts, cut into small pieces

½ cup diced red onion

8 cups zucchini "pasta" (see page 100)

¼ cup hemp seeds

2 tbsp sunflower seeds

2 tbsp chopped fresh parsley or cilantro

2 tbsp chopped fresh basil

½ tsp grated organic lime zest

Optional garnishes: 2 tbsp sprouts of choice or 1 Vietnamese chili pepper, finely diced, with seeds for extra heat

In a small bowl, combine 2 tbsp olive oil, rice vinegar, lime juice, brown sugar, fish sauce, scallions, and 1 tbsp minced garlic. Stir and set aside.

In a medium skillet, heat 1 tbsp olive oil over medium-high heat. Add chicken, red onion, and remaining garlic. Cook, stirring, for 8 minutes, until chicken is no longer pink. Transfer to a bowl.

Add the remaining 1 tbsp olive oil and then the zucchini pasta to skillet and stir-fry for 2 minutes. Stir in scallion mixture. Divide among 4 plates and top with cooked chicken mixture.

Combine hemp seeds, sunflower seeds, parsley or cilantro, basil, and lime zest in a bowl and sprinkle on pad Thai. Top with sprouts or chili pepper, if desired.

Note: Uncooked sprouts can lead to serious food-borne illnesses. You can always sauté to offset any potential dangers.

Makes 4 servings

HEALTHY CHICKEN PARMESAN

For crispy chicken breasts, dredge the pounded breasts in panko bread crumbs before cooking. **Note:** You don't need to use egg as a batter for the chicken if you use chicken with skin. Using an egg batter will make the dish more reactive.

  2 boneless chicken breasts
  2 tbsp extra virgin olive oil
  ½ cup Low-Reactive Tomato Sauce (page 137)
  ¼ cup grated goat-cheese Gouda or Cheddar
  Optional: chopped fresh basil, rosemary, oregano, or thyme

If chicken breasts are uneven, pound with a mallet to an even thickness. Heat oil in a cast-iron skillet over medium heat. Add chicken breasts and cook for 8 minutes. Turn broiler on high. Turn chicken over and cook in pan for an additional 4 minutes. Top chicken with tomato sauce and cheese and place under broiler for 2 to 3 minutes to get a nice crispy browned cheese topping. If you like, top with herbs of choice.

Makes 2 servings

SPICY CHICKEN AND POTATO STEW
(*TAK TORITANG*)

The Plan version of *tak toritang* switches out *gochujang,* a traditional Korean hot sauce, as we find it slightly more reactive than Sriracha. Most people tolerate small amounts of potatoes very well when mixed with copious amounts of other vegetables!

Red potatoes contain less starch than other potatoes, such as baking potatoes, making them less reactive. You can make this in a soup pot in less time, but there is something that is so great about throwing everything in a slow cooker and coming home to a hearty, warm dinner. **Note:** Molasses is very rich in iron!

8 bone-in chicken thighs

2 small red potatoes, chopped

4 carrots, chopped

1 large onion, chopped

2 cups chopped deveined kale

4 cloves garlic, chopped

2-inch piece fresh ginger, peeled and grated (about 1 tbsp)

2 cups low-sodium or homemade chicken stock

2 cups water

¼ cup rice cooking wine

4 tbsp Sriracha

1 tsp rice vinegar (natural, not seasoned)

1 tsp honey

2 tsp molasses (or substitute 2 tsp more honey)

¼ tsp sea salt

Dash of cayenne pepper

Combine all ingredients in a slow cooker and cook on high for 6 to 8 hours.

Makes 4 to 6 servings

SWEET AND SOUR CHICKEN

¼ cup rice vinegar (natural, not seasoned)

¼ cup Spicy Apricot Sauce (page 145)

Juice of 1 lime (1½ to 2 tbsp)

½ tsp sea salt

2 tbsp extra virgin olive oil

1 lb skinless boneless chicken breasts cut into bite-sized pieces

4 cloves garlic, minced

2 tsp finely grated peeled fresh ginger

2 cups low-sodium or homemade chicken stock

2 cups chopped broccoli

2 cups chopped zucchini

2 cups chopped deveined kale

½ cup chopped shiitake or enoki mushrooms

¼ cup chopped canned water chestnuts (citric acid–free)

Whisk rice vinegar, apricot sauce, lime juice, and salt in a small bowl. Set aside.

Heat 1 tbsp olive oil in a large skillet over medium-high heat. Add chicken and cook for 2 minutes. Transfer to a plate. Add remaining 1 tbsp oil, garlic, and ginger to pan and cook, stirring, for 30 seconds. Add stock and bring to a boil, stirring constantly. Add chicken, along with broccoli, zucchini, kale, and mushrooms. Reduce heat to a simmer, cover, and cook for 8 to 10 minutes, until chicken is cooked through. Add water chestnuts and apricot sauce mixture. Stir well, cooking for an additional minute.

Makes 4 servings

CHICKEN WITH ITALIAN HERBS
AND ORANGE ZEST

Dried Italian herbs

4 chicken thighs or 2 breasts

2 tbsp organic orange zest

Oil for pan

Preheat oven to 350°F.

Liberally sprinkle Italian herbs on chicken so each breast is covered. Sprinkle with orange zest. Place chicken in an oiled cast-iron skillet and bake for 20 to 30 minutes, depending on the thickness of the breasts, until cooked through.

Makes 2 servings

PANKO-CRUSTED CHICKEN TENDERS

We love chicken thighs in our family because they are so much juicier than breasts! But no matter your preference, both cuts will work well with this recipe and offer great nutrition and nutrients.

1 lb boneless chicken breast or thighs

¾ cup panko bread crumbs or gluten-free panko

4 tbsp extra virgin olive oil

Cut chicken into 1-inch strips. Put panko in a shallow bowl, add the chicken, and press down making sure each side is well coated.

Heat 2 tbsp olive oil in a skillet over medium heat and swirl to coat bottom of pan. Add chicken and cook 6 to 8 minutes, until browned on bottom. Use tongs to turn over and add remaining 2 tbsp extra virgin olive oil. Cook chicken until cooked through, 8 to 10 more minutes.

Note: Instead of pan frying, you can bake the chicken on a baking sheet at 375°F for 20 to 25 minutes.

Makes 2 to 4 servings

BUTTERNUT SQUASH–CHICKEN "TOSTADAS"

1 medium butternut squash

4 tbsp extra virgin olive oil

1 red onion, chopped

1 jalapeño pepper, chopped

2 cloves garlic, minced

1 tsp chipotle powder, or to taste

Dash of sea salt

2 chicken thighs, cooked, meat removed from bone, and diced

2 tbsp Low-Reactive Tomato Sauce (page 137)

Juice of 1 lime (about 2 tbsp)

1 cup chopped romaine lettuce

½ cup Plan Guacamole (page 114) or avocado chunks

Cut off top of squash and slice flesh into 16 (¼-inch-thick) rounds. Heat 2 tbsp olive oil in a skillet and cook squash until browned, 3 minutes per side. These will be your shells for the "tostadas."

Heat the remaining 2 tbsp olive oil in a medium pan. Add onion, jalapeño, garlic, chipotle powder, and salt and sauté for 2 to 3 minutes, until browned. Transfer to a large bowl and stir in diced chicken, tomato sauce, and lime juice.

Top butternut squash rounds with chicken mixture and then top with lettuce and guacamole to make your open-face taco.

Makes 4 servings

ROAST CHICKEN

Cooking in cast-iron skillets boosts the iron content of your meal!

1 whole chicken, 3 to 4 lbs, neck and giblets removed from cavity

2 tbsp extra virgin olive oil

1 tsp sea salt

Freshly ground black pepper

Optional: 1 medium lemon, thinly sliced

Optional: 1 bunch fresh dill and 1 bunch fresh parsley, chopped

Preheat oven to 425°F and arrange a rack in the middle. Rinse chicken under cold water and pat dry with paper towels. Drizzle olive oil on the chicken and rub it all over the skin. Season all over with salt and pepper. If using, place lemon and herbs inside cavity.

Place the chicken, breast side up, in a cast-iron skillet or roasting pan. Roast for 15 minutes. Reduce temperature to 400°F and continue roasting until juices run clear and a thermometer inserted into the inner thigh (but not touching bone) registers 165°F, 50 to 60 minutes. The chicken should have a nice brown crust. Remove chicken from oven and let rest 10 to 15 minutes before serving. Use remaining chicken jus for chicken broth.

Makes 4 to 8 servings

WHOLE CHICKEN IN A SLOW COOKER

A busy person's delight, this chicken is so moist and tender you won't believe it.

2 tsp dried sage

1 tsp dried rosemary

1 tsp dried tarragon

1 tsp garlic powder

¼ tsp cayenne

½ tsp salt

½ tsp freshly ground black pepper

1 whole chicken, 3 to 4 lbs, neck and giblets removed from cavity

1 lemon, sliced

6 cloves garlic, peeled

1½ cups chopped fennel

2 large Spanish onions, cut into large chunks

2 tbsp extra virgin olive oil

Combine herbs and spices in a small bowl. Rub mixture all over chicken. Place lemon slices, garlic, and ½ cup fennel inside chicken cavity. Place onions and the remaining fennel on the bottom of a slow cooker and drizzle with olive oil. Place seasoned chicken on top of onions, cover, and cook for 4 to 5 hours on high.

Makes 8 servings

CORNISH GAME HENS

It's a family tradition to serve a Cornish game hen for each person at our Thanksgiving dinner—it's much less reactive than turkey!

4 lemons

15 cloves garlic, peeled

¼ cup fresh parsley leaves

2 tbsp dried rosemary

2 tbsp dried thyme

2 tbsp dried sage

2 tsp lemon juice

1 tsp coarse sea salt

1 tsp freshly ground black pepper, plus more for sprinkling

3 tbsp extra virgin olive oil, plus more for greasing

4 Cornish game hens

Preheat oven to 400°F.

Trim ends from lemons, cut into wedges, and seed. Chop 3 of the garlic cloves. Set aside the remaining whole garlic cloves with the lemon wedges.

Place the chopped garlic, parsley, rosemary, thyme, sage, lemon juice, salt, pepper, and 3 tbsp olive oil in a food processor. Blend.

Loosen skin from hens. Put 3 to 4 tbsp of herb mixture under the skin of each hen. Place hens in a lightly greased cast-iron skillet and stuff each with 1 lemon and 3 cloves of garlic. Roast for 50 minutes, or until a meat thermometer reads 165°F when inserted into a thigh. Let sit 10 to 15 minutes before serving.

Makes 4 servings

DUCK BREAST TACOS

1 duck breast

¼ cup chopped mango

1 roasted jalapeño pepper

¼ cup chopped fresh cilantro or parsley

2 cloves garlic, peeled

2 tbsp fresh lime juice

2 tbsp extra virgin olive oil

8 Veg Chia Crisps (page 120) or 4 Flour Tortillas (page 121)

1 large carrot, grated

½ small beet, grated

½ cup goat-cheese ricotta or grated goat-cheese Cheddar

Preheat oven to 350°F.

Score breast skin by making an X in it until you see flesh below.

Heat a small cast-iron skillet over medium heat. Add duck breast, fat side down, and cook until skin is golden brown, about 10 minutes; pour off fat as it accumulates in pan. You can transfer fat to a bowl for later use. Transfer skillet to oven and roast breast for about 10 minutes, until a meat thermometer inserted into thickest part registers 135°F. Let duck rest for 5 minutes.

Combine mango, jalapeño, cilantro or parsley, garlic, and lime juice in a food processor and pulse until cilantro is finely chopped. Add olive oil and puree until fairly smooth.

Slice duck into ⅛-inch-thin slices. Layer crackers with duck, carrot, beet, goat cheese, and top with mango-jalapeño sauce.

Optional: Remove and discard skin before adding mango.

Makes 2 to 3 servings

PAN-SEARED CINNAMON DUCK BREASTS
WITH BALSAMIC JUS

1 large clove garlic, finely chopped

1-inch piece fresh ginger, peeled and grated (about 1 tbsp)

2 tsp ground cinnamon

½ tsp ground cumin

½ tsp cardamom

½ tsp cayenne

1 tsp sea salt

½ tsp freshly ground black pepper

4 duck breasts

¼ cup dry red wine

2 tbsp balsamic vinegar

Combine garlic, ginger, cinnamon, cumin, cardamom, cayenne, salt, and pepper in a large bowl and mix well. Add duck breasts and turn to coat. Cover and refrigerate for at least 1 hour or up to 24 hours.

Remove duck from refrigerator 1 hour before cooking. Score breast skins by making an X in skin until you see flesh below.

Preheat oven to 400°F. Heat a large cast-iron skillet over medium-high heat for 2 minutes. Add duck breasts, skin side down, and sear for 5 minutes; turn and sear for 5 minutes on other sides. Transfer pan to oven and roast duck for 5 minutes, until a meat thermometer inserted into the thickest part registers 135°F. Transfer duck breasts to a plate and keep warm.

To make the balsamic jus, pour off fat from pan. Return pan to medium-high heat, add wine, and stir to scrape up browned bits from bottom of pan. Simmer until wine is reduced by half. Add balsamic vinegar and cook to reduce for several more minutes. Cut duck breasts into thin diagonal slices and serve drizzled with balsamic jus.

Makes 6 to 8 servings

VENISON MEDALLIONS IN APPLE BOURBON SAUCE

2 venison medallions (6 to 8 oz each)
¼ tsp sea salt
Freshly ground black pepper, to taste
2 tbsp extra virgin olive oil
Apple Bourbon Sauce (page 147)

Season venison on both sides with salt and pepper. In a large skillet, heat oil over medium-high heat. Add venison and cook, 3 to 4 minutes per side for medium-rare. Serve with Apple Bourbon Sauce.

Note: All game is best cooked rare to medium-rare because game and wild meat have a higher omega-3 content than conventionally raised meat.

Makes 2 servings

LAMB SHEPHERD'S PIE

This filling dish is a true Planner Thanksgiving tradition.

  1 lb ground lamb

  1 onion, chopped

  3 cloves garlic, minced

  1 tsp ground cinnamon

  1 tsp cayenne

  1 tsp ground cumin

  ½ tsp nutmeg

  1 zucchini, chopped into 1-inch cubes

  1 head kale, deveined and chopped

  1 medium potato, cut into 1-inch cubes

  1 medium butternut squash, cut into 1-inch cubes

  ½ cup (1 stick) unsalted butter, softened

  ½ cup canned full-fat unsweetened coconut milk

  Optional: 1 tsp dried sage or other herbs of choice

  ¼ tsp coarse grain sea salt

Preheat oven to 400°F.

Heat a large skillet over medium heat. Add lamb, onion, garlic, and spices and cook, stirring, until lamb is browned, about 6 minutes. Add zucchini and cook 5 minutes. Add kale, cover, and remove from heat. Let steam for 5 to 6 minutes, until kale is thoroughly cooked. Stir when done.

Meanwhile, in a steamer basket set in a large pot with 1 inch of simmering water, layer the potato cubes, then top with the squash cubes. Steam for about 8 minutes, until tender. Transfer potatoes and squash to two separate bowls. Add half the butter and coconut milk to potatoes and half to the squash. Mash each until creamy. Season with sage or other herbs, if desired, and salt.

Layer a 10x10-inch casserole dish with the mashed potatoes, then the lamb-kale mixture, and then the mashed squash. Bake for 15 minutes, until top is crispy brown.

Makes 6 servings

LAMB BURGERS

Our famous lamb burgers, modified with onions instead of shiitakes to lower cost and up the flavor! These are crowd-pleasers.

    1 lb ground lamb
    1 zucchini, grated
    ¼ cup chopped red onion
    Optional: herbs of choice such as herbes de Provence or salt-free Italian herb blend
    Optional: 4 shiitake mushrooms, finely chopped (for extra chewy texture)
    Oil for pan

Combine all ingredients except oil in a bowl. Form into 4 patties. Heat an oiled medium skillet over medium heat. Add the patties to the skillet and cook, turning once, until medium-rare, 6 to 8 minutes.

Makes 4 servings

LAMB AND APRICOT TAGINE

Lamb shoulder is an inexpensive cut that is very rich and flavorful, and is enhanced by these flavorful spices.

    ¼ cup extra virgin olive oil

    2 lb lamb shoulder, cut into 2- or 3-inch pieces

    ½ tsp salt

    Freshly ground black pepper, to taste

    2 medium onions, grated or very finely chopped

    3 cloves garlic, pressed or finely chopped

    2 tbsp Spicy Baharat Rub (page 142)

    ½ tsp turmeric

    1 cinnamon stick

    ¼ cup Carrot Ginger Soup (page 101)

    1 cup low-sodium or homemade vegetarian stock or Carrot Soup Essence (page 102)

    1 cup dried apricots, chopped

    1 tbsp honey

    1 tsp ground cinnamon

    Optional: ¼ cup almond slivers

Heat oil in a large heavy pot over medium-high heat. Season lamb with salt and pepper. Add lamb to pot and brown all over, 3 to 4 minutes per side. Transfer lamb to a medium bowl.

Add onions to pot; reduce heat to medium and sauté until soft and beginning to turn golden, about 5 minutes. Add garlic, spice rub, turmeric, and cinnamon stick and sauté for 1 minute. Add carrot ginger soup, return lamb to pot, and bring to a simmer. Add stock or soup essence, reduce heat to low, and simmer for 1 hour, until lamb is tender. Discard cinnamon stick. Add apricots, honey, and ground cinnamon. Stir well and simmer for an additional 10 minutes. Serve in separate bowls and top with almonds, if desired.

Makes 6 to 8 servings

MEDITERRANEAN GRILLED LAMB CHOPS

Summer is a great time to put all of your garden or windowsill herbs to work in this delicious recipe! You can use the chop of your choice. Shoulder has a richer lamb taste. Rib or loin is more mild and closer to beef in flavor.

¼ cup extra virgin olive oil, plus more for oiling the grate

2 cloves garlic, minced

1 tbsp minced fresh rosemary

1 tsp minced fresh oregano

½ tsp minced fresh thyme

⅛ tsp sea salt

½ tsp freshly ground black pepper

4 lamb chops, 6 to 8 oz each

Optional: ½ cup Hemp Seed Pesto (page 140) for basting

Preheat grill for high heat and lightly oil the grate, or heat broiler.

In a shallow dish, combine ¼ cup oil with garlic, rosemary, oregano, thyme, salt, and pepper. Add lamb chops and turn to coat. Let marinate 20 minutes.

Grill or broil lamb chops on one side for 6 to 7 minutes. Baste with hemp pesto, if desired. Turn and cook until done, 2 to 3 minutes longer.

Makes 2 to 4 servings

MAMA'S MINI LAMB MEATBALLS

Growing up in New York City I knew I had a tough job ahead if I were to come up with a meatball recipe that would stand muster. I knew the recipe worked when I had my Sicilian friends ask how I made them, and best of all? Brayden *loves* them!

Extra virgin olive oil for the baking sheet

1 lb ground lamb

¼ cup Low-Reactive Tomato Sauce (page 137)

¼ cup panko bread crumbs or gluten-free panko

Preheat oven to 375°F. Grease a baking sheet. Combine all ingredients in a mixing bowl. Form into 2-inch round meatballs and arrange on prepared sheet. Bake for 15 minutes for medium-well.

Makes 4 servings (12 meatballs)

GROUND BEEF MOLE

1 medium white onion, diced

2 to 3 cloves garlic, minced

2 tsp chipotle powder

2 tsp cocoa powder

1 tsp ground cinnamon

½ tsp ground cloves

½ tsp ground cumin

Sea salt and freshly ground black pepper, to taste

1 lb ground beef

Extra virgin olive oil

3 cups chopped deveined kale

1 cup julienne carrots

1 cup julienne zucchini

In a medium bowl add onion, garlic, and spices to the burger. Mix thoroughly and let marinate for at least 30 minutes and up to 24 hours in the refrigerator. Heat a large oiled skillet, add the beef, and sauté for 2 minutes. Remove beef from pan and set aside in a dish. Add kale, carrots, and zucchini to the pan and cook until tender, 7 to 10 minutes. Add beef and cook for 2 minutes for medium, 5 or 6 minutes for well done.

Note: The mole is delicious served with Veg Chia Crisps (page 120), Plan Guacamole (page 114), and grated goat-cheese Cheddar.

Makes 4 servings

BEEF CARPACCIO

On hot summer nights you often want to have a simple light dish and beef carpaccio fits the bill when it's mixed with fresh summer greens. Raw meat may contain harmful bacteria, including *salmonella, listeria, campylobacter,* and *E. coli,* that can cause foodborne illness, so make sure to check with your butcher and find the highest quality meat available approved for consumption without cooking.

   8 oz beef tenderloin, from the tip end of the roast

   6 cups baby romaine or greens of choice

   1 cup chopped radicchio

   ¼ cup Oregano Garlic Vinaigrette (page 150)

   Freshly ground black pepper, to taste

   Shaved pecorino (about 2 oz)

Wrap tenderloin in plastic wrap and place in the freezer for 1 hour. Slice beef into thin (about ¼-inch-thick) slices. Sandwich slices between plastic wrap or wax paper and use a mallet to pound into thinner slices.

Season baby romaine or other greens and radicchio with vinaigrette and freshly ground black pepper. Top salad with beef and shaved pecorino.

Makes 2 servings

STEAK FAJITAS

There's no way you should eat fajitas alone! This recipe, perfect for entertaining, serves 8 to 10 very well. I like my fajitas very rare and only cook them for one minute. Explore what works best for your taste!

    2 tbsp lime juice

    1 tsp ground cumin

    1 tsp chipotle powder

    ½ tsp sea salt

    1 tsp black pepper

    4 tbsp extra virgin olive oil

    2 lb skirt steak, trimmed and cut into 1-inch strips

    2 medium red onions, thinly sliced

    4 garlic cloves, chopped

    3 zucchini, cut into strips

Combine lime juice, cumin, chipotle, sea salt, black pepper, and 2 tbsp of olive oil in a large bowl and whisk. Add steak, onions, garlic cloves, and zucchini and mix well. Cover and marinate in refrigerator for 2 hours or up to 24 hours.

Heat remaining 2 tbsp olive oil in a large skillet over medium heat. Add beef and vegetables in two batches and cook to desired doneness.

Note: This works well when served with Chipotle-Avo Dressing (page 151) and lettuce, with grated cheese on the side.

Makes 8 to 10 servings

SPICY ORANGE BEEF

I've made this dish with every cut of beef from leftover steak to fajitas or skirt.

    Zest of 1 organic orange

    1 tbsp rice vinegar (natural, not seasoned)

    1 tsp honey or agave nectar

    ¼ tsp coarse grain sea salt

2 tbsp extra virgin olive oil

1 lb beef, cut into ½-inch pieces for stir-fry

3 cloves garlic, chopped

1-inch piece fresh ginger, peeled and chopped (about 1 tbsp)

1 tsp crushed red pepper flakes

3 cups broccoli florets

½ cup sliced scallion greens

Combine zest, rice vinegar, honey or agave, and salt in a bowl and stir to combine. Heat 1 tbsp olive oil in a skillet over medium-high heat. Add beef and stir-fry for 1 minute. Transfer beef to a plate and set aside. Add remaining 1 tbsp olive oil to pan. Add garlic, ginger, and crushed red pepper flakes and stir-fry for about 30 seconds. Add broccoli and cook for 4 minutes, until broccoli is tender. Add orange zest mixture, beef, and scallions and stir-fry for an additional 2 to 3 minutes, until beef is medium-rare.

Makes 4 servings

PRIME RIB

This is a dish fit for a king, and you'll probably still have some leftovers, too! Remember, most beef is best when cooked medium-rare. A classic dish for large family gatherings.

10-lb beef rib roast

10 cloves garlic, chopped

¼ cup extra virgin olive oil

2 tsp dried thyme

2 tsp dried sage

2 tsp dried rosemary

2 tsp sea salt

2 tsp freshly ground black pepper

Place beef roast in a roasting pan with fatty side up. In a small bowl, mix together garlic, oil, thyme, sage, rosemary, salt, and pepper. Drizzle over roast and let marinate about 2 hours at room temperature. (This is very important as the meat needs to be at room temperature so the roast cooks evenly.)

Preheat oven to 475°F.

Put roast in oven and roast for 15 minutes. Turn oven down to 325°F and roast until meat thermometer inserted in thickest part of roast reads 120°F for medium-rare (see Note). This will take about 15 minutes per pound, or 2½ hours for a 10-lb roast. Every ½ hour, baste the cut ends of the roast with the fat accumulated in the roasting pan. Do not cover roast.

Transfer to a large platter, tent loosely with foil, and let rest for 30 minutes before serving, to keep juices intact.

Note: If you prefer your roast rare, remove it at 110°F; for medium, at 130°F.

Makes 20 servings

ROMAN-STYLE STEAK

½ cup extra virgin olive oil, plus more for oiling the grate

2 large garlic cloves, finely chopped

1 tbsp finely chopped fresh rosemary

2 rib-eye steaks (about 6 oz each), 1-inch thick

Dash of sea salt

Freshly ground black pepper, to taste

Optional: 1 tbsp balsamic vinegar

In a food processor, combine olive oil, garlic, and rosemary and pulse for 1 minute. Place steaks in a shallow baking dish; rub both sides with salt and pepper and coat with garlic-rosemary mixture. Cover with plastic wrap and marinate at least 30 minutes at room temperature, or up to 1 day in refrigerator, turning once or twice.

If steaks are refrigerated, let them come to room temperature for up to 2 hours before cooking. Preheat grill for medium-high heat and lightly oil the grate, or preheat broiler and place rack 4 to 6 inches from heat source.

Remove steaks from marinade and pat dry with paper towels. Grill or broil, turning once, until done to taste, about 4 minutes on each side for medium-rare. Serve immediately. Drizzle with balsamic vinegar, if desired.

Makes 2 servings

Desserts

Dessert is a pleasure that can be a routine part of The Plan. You're probably thinking, "Hold on a minute! Aren't sugar and chocolate and sweets bad for you?" Well, if you're living off 1,200 calories a day, yes, they can be. When you have such minimal food intake, you're just not getting enough nutrients, fats, and proteins to offset the sugar! But if you're eating a vitamin- and mineral-rich diet, which just happens to have you eating 2,000 to 3,000 calories a day like The Plan, you can see how this is a completely different story! Makes sense, right? That's why one of my favorite desserts to plug in as an afternoon snack is my red velvet cupcake! When you follow The Plan, you are keeping your insulin and yeast in check and sweets really are fine in moderation. And when you're eating according to The Plan and providing your body with the nutrients it needs, that's exactly how you'll want to have sweets—in moderation. Sugar shouldn't be the boss of you! It helps that Plan desserts are rich in fiber, good fats, and protein. The proteins will help to keep your blood sugar stable and the fat will slow down the absorption of the sugar.

And what is the best fat to have in desserts? Butter, of course! I know what you're thinking: "Butter? Isn't butter bad for you? What about cholesterol?" Breathe a sigh of relief. Cholesterol is not the villain; in fact it's necessary for the formation of cell membranes which protect our bodies from invaders. Our cell walls have a phospholipid barrier, which means that fats help to stabilize our cell walls. When our body senses that inflammation is increasing and our cell walls are becoming unstable, it produces extra cholesterol, a lipid, to step in and help provide stability so we aren't susceptible to attack.

So it's not the cholesterol we need to be concerned about, but the source of inflammation that's causing your body to elevate its cholesterol levels. High cholesterol is essentially a marker of inflammation. Find your reactive foods, eliminate them from your diet, and your cholesterol lowers. We see Planners with high cholesterol lower their cholesterol levels quickly and dramatically on The Plan. Women drop an average of 40 plus points in a month and men drop an average of 60 points. So remember, inflammatory foods raise cholesterol. Butter will raise your cholesterol if you are reactive to it, just like asparagus will raise your cholesterol if you're reactive to it.

So don't stress about helping yourself to dessert, especially any of the nutrient-dense and delicious desserts in this chapter. I hope you enjoy these desserts as much as my family does!

What's Better than Butter?

In addition to being delicious, butter is chock-full of goodness:

Vitamin A: essential for thyroid and adrenal health, powerful antioxidant
Vitamin E: essential for heart health, diabetes management, fighting cancer, and balancing hormones
Selenium: essential for thyroid health, immune system
Lecithin: necessary for proper assimilation of cholesterol and liver function
Lauric acid: combats yeast
Vitamin D: necessary for calcium absorption, heart health, and skin conditions
Iodine: essential for thyroid health

What About Coconut Oil?

Our savvy Planners have asked about coconut oil, a popular ingredient in many paleo recipes. (In case it's new to you, paleo is a dietary protocol that's meant to re-create the way ancient man would have eaten.) I have found coconut oil to be about 18 percent reactive and it will cause weight stabilization instead of weight loss. Now 18 percent is pretty good odds that you won't have an issue, but I want you to be sure that a food works for you before you make it a mainstay in your diet!

ROSE WATER–CHOCOLATE MACAROONS

Macaroons

2 cups shredded unsweetened coconut

2 tbsp agave nectar

2 tbsp chia seeds

1 tsp pure vanilla extract

1 tsp rose water

Chocolate Glaze

½ cup chocolate chips or chopped chocolate

2 tbsp Silk coconut milk or Rice Dream

For macaroons, line a baking sheet with wax paper or parchment paper.

Combine all ingredients in a food processor and blend well. Let sit for 10 minutes. Form dough into about 16 (2-inch) balls and arrange on prepared baking sheet. Place in the freezer for a half hour.

For glaze, combine chocolate and coconut milk or Rice Dream in a small saucepan over low heat. Stir frequently until chocolate melts, 2 to 3 minutes. Transfer to a measuring cup.

Remove macaroons from freezer and lightly drizzle chocolate on top of each one. Refrigerate for at least 20 minutes to set before serving. Serve chilled or at room temperature.

Makes 16 macaroons

TALIA'S GLUTEN-FREE COOKIES

Talia is a lovely little girl who was miserable with not being able to eat her favorite desserts because of gluten sensitivity. I had her try a bunch of recipes and this was her favorite. I think someday we might have a stellar gluten-free baker named Talia.

1 cup raw almond butter

½ cup agave nectar

¼ cup avocado

¼ cup packed brown sugar

4 tbsp cocoa powder

½ tsp pure vanilla extract

¼ tsp baking soda

2 tbsp confectioners' sugar, for topping

Combine almond butter, agave, avocado, brown sugar, 2 tbsp cocoa, vanilla, and baking soda in a large bowl and mix well with a hand mixer. Refrigerate dough for 20 to 30 minutes.

Preheat oven to 350°F.

Form chilled dough into 16 to 20 (1-inch) balls and arrange on an ungreased baking sheet. Bake 8 to 10 minutes, until golden brown. Let cool.

For topping, mix remaining cocoa and confectioners' sugar together in a small bowl. Once cookies are cooled, roll balls in cocoa-sugar mix. Serve and enjoy.

Makes 16 to 20 cookies

THANKSGIVING MINI MUFFINS

1 cup cooked butternut squash or canned pumpkin

⅓ cup (⅔ stick) unsalted butter, softened, plus more for greasing

4 large eggs, well beaten

¼ cup honey

½ cup coconut flour

1 tsp pure vanilla extract

½ tsp nutmeg

½ tsp cardamom

⅛ tsp ground cloves

⅛ tsp baking soda

Preheat oven to 350°F. Butter a 12-cup mini muffin tin.

Combine all ingredients in a food processor and blend for 1 minute. Scrape sides to integrate all ingredients. Blend for an additional minute, until mixture thickens.

Fill muffin cups evenly with batter. Bake for 10 to 12 minutes. Insert a toothpick to determine if they're done. Serve warm.

Makes 12 muffins

CARROT CAKE

2 cups all-purpose flour, plus more for the pan

¼ cup (½ stick) unsalted butter, softened, plus more for greasing

4 cups grated carrots (4 to 5 medium carrots)

½ cup agave nectar

2 large eggs

2 tbsp chia seeds

2 tsp ground cinnamon

1 tsp nutmeg

½ tsp baking soda

¼ tsp salt

Optional: Goat Cheese Icing (page 191)

Preheat oven to 350°F. Grease and flour a 9x13-inch baking pan.

Combine all ingredients (except icing) in a large bowl or food processor. Mix well with a hand blender or food processor.

Transfer batter to prepared pan. Bake for 40 minutes; insert a toothpick to determine doneness. If icing the cake, let it cool slightly first. Otherwise, serve warm or at room temperature.

Makes 8 to 10 servings

RED VELVET CUPCAKES WITH GOAT CHEESE ICING

This protein-rich dessert could work for a breakfast or a snack if you leave off the icing. Keep the icing, and it is my stepdaughter's favorite dessert.

Goat Cheese Icing

1½ cups confectioners' sugar

4 oz goat cheese

¼ cup (½ stick) unsalted butter, softened

1 tsp pure vanilla extract

Red Velvet Cupcakes

½ cup (1 stick) unsalted butter, softened, plus more for greasing

1 large beet, cut into 1-inch cubes

½ cup agave nectar or honey

3 large eggs

2 tsp pure vanilla extract

3½ cups blanched almond flour

⅓ cup cocoa powder

¼ tsp baking soda

For icing, combine all ingredients in a food processor and blend for 1 minute. Place in a small bowl, cover, and chill in the refrigerator while you make the cupcakes.

For cupcakes, preheat oven to 350°F. Butter a 12-cup muffin tin.

Cook cubed beet in a pot of boiling water for 20 minutes, until completely softened. Run under cold water until completely cooled. (You should have about 2 cups.)

Combine beet, agave or honey, ½ cup softened butter, eggs, and vanilla in food processor and blend for 2 minutes, until ingredients are completely combined. Add almond flour, cocoa, and baking soda and mix completely. Batter will feel very moist, but ignore the inclination to add more almond flour!

Divide batter evenly among the 12 buttered muffin cups. Bake for 18 minutes, until a toothpick inserted in centers comes out clean. Let cool completely before frosting with the icing.

Makes 12 cupcakes

ALMOND FLOUR PIE DOUGH

This delicious pie crust is the perfect match for our Plan-friendly Pumpkin Pie (page 193) and Raw Pecan Pie (below).

1½ cups almond flour

¼ cup (½ stick) unsalted butter, softened

2 tsp honey

1 tsp pure vanilla extract

½ tsp ground cinnamon

½ tsp cardamom

Place all ingredients in a food processor and blend. Combine dough into a ball. The dough will keep, covered, for 2 days in the refrigerator.

Preheat oven to 350°F. Roll dough out between 2 sheets of wax paper. Fit dough into an 8-inch springform pan.

Bake pie crust for 8 to 10 minutes, until it is lightly browned.

Makes 1 (8-inch) pie shell

RAW PECAN PIE

1½ cups raw pecans, plus more for garnish

1 cup applesauce

½ cup chia seeds

2 tsp pure vanilla extract

1 tbsp ground cinnamon

⅛ tsp nutmeg

Almond Flour Pie Dough (above), prebaked

Combine pecans, applesauce, chia seeds, vanilla, cinnamon, and nutmeg in a food processor. Blend until smooth, stopping to scrape down the sides periodically. Pour filling evenly over crust. Top with additional pecans—decorate as you desire. Cover and freeze for at least 3 to 4 hours or overnight. Remove from freezer, cut, and serve.

Makes 8 servings

PUMPKIN PIE

3 cups cooked pumpkin

2 large eggs

¾ cup Silk coconut milk or Rice Dream

2 tbsp brown sugar

1 tsp pure vanilla extract

1 tsp ground cinnamon

½ tsp allspice

½ tsp nutmeg

Almond Flour Pie Dough (page 192) or regular pre-made pie crust

Preheat oven to 375°F.

Combine pumpkin, eggs, coconut milk or Rice Dream, brown sugar, vanilla, cinnamon, allspice, and nutmeg in a food processor and blend until smooth. Pour into pie shell. Bake for 50 minutes, until toothpick comes out clean. Let cool on a wire rack for 10 minutes before serving.

Makes 8 servings

SO RICH YOU COULD DIE CHOCOLATE PIE

12 oz Valrhona chocolate, finely chopped; or 12 oz semisweet chocolate chips

1 cup heavy whipping cream

½ cup Silk Coconut milk or Rice Dream

1 tsp vanilla

Almond Flour Pie Dough (page 192), prebaked

Optional: Katie's Whipped Coconut Cream (page 194) or Pear Ice Cream (page 194), to serve

Combine chocolate, whipping cream, and coconut milk or Rice Dream in a medium bowl and microwave for 1 minute. Stir to blend and then microwave for another 1 minute. Stir until smooth. Stir in vanilla.

Pour chocolate filling into pie shell and chill in refrigerator for 2 hours, until firm to the touch. If you like, serve with fresh whipped cream or pear ice cream.

Note: Add shredded coconut or almond slivers to the pie crust dough.

Makes 10 to 12 servings

KATIE'S WHIPPED COCONUT CREAM

Our wonderful Dr. Katie developed this dairy-free version of whipped cream so our lactose-intolerant friends don't have to miss out on a wonderful dessert topping.

1 (14-oz) can full-fat unsweetened coconut milk

Optional: 1 to 2 tbsp agave nectar

Optional: 1 tsp pure vanilla extract

Chill the can of coconut milk in the fridge for 8 hours or overnight.

Open the can without shaking it. Separate the cream on top from the liquid and transfer to a large bowl; discard the liquid. Add agave and vanilla to cream, if desired. Using a hand or stand mixer, whip coconut until it forms creamy peaks, about 3 minutes. Serve immediately.

Makes 4 to 6 servings

PEAR ICE CREAM

Simple and refreshing, feel free to sub in any fruit that works for your chemistry!

1 cup chopped cored pear

¾ cup canned full-fat unsweetened coconut milk

Optional: Cinnamon to taste

Special equipment: 2 to 4 (4-oz) mason jars

Place pear in freezer for at least 2 hours. Combine frozen pear, coconut milk, and cinnamon, if desired, in blender and blend well. Spoon into individual mason jars and freeze for 1 hour. Serve immediately.

Makes 2 to 4 servings

FROZEN RICOTTA COOKIE SANDWICHES

One of my favorite ways to utilize the lavender I grow. Lemon verbena works wonderfully, too!

1 cup fresh goat-cheese ricotta

1 cup confectioners' sugar

1 tsp pure vanilla extract

1 tsp dried lavender flowers

16 graham cracker squares (from 8 sheets)

Line a baking sheet with wax paper. In a food processor, combine ricotta, confectioners' sugar, vanilla, and lavender, and blend well. Using an ice cream scooper, scoop mixture into 8 balls and place on prepared baking sheet. Place sheet in freezer for several hours, until ricotta balls are frozen.

Sandwich frozen ricotta between graham crackers immediately before serving.

Makes 8 servings

WATERMELON LIME POPS

Both watermelon and lime are great natural diuretics, perfect for hot summer days!

2 cups cubed watermelon

2 tbsp lime juice

2 tbsp honey

Combine watermelon, lime juice, and honey in a blender and blend until smooth. Pour into 4 ice pop molds and insert sticks. Freeze for 5 hours or longer.

Makes 4 pops

INDIAN CHEESE DESSERT (*RAS MALAI*)

Ras Malai is truly one of my favorite desserts. I had it for the first time in New York City's Little India about thirty years ago and instantly fell in love. The subtle scent and taste of rose is divine!

2 cups goat ricotta or raw milk ricotta

½ cup honey

3 cups Silk coconut milk or Rice Dream

½ tsp cardamom

1 tsp rose water

¼ cup almond slivers

Preheat oven to 350°F. Line a 12-cup muffin tin with paper liners.

Blend ricotta and honey together in a food processor. Use an ice cream scoop to evenly scoop ricotta mixture into the 12 lined muffin cups. Bake for 30 to 35 minutes, until firm to the touch. Let ricotta cheese balls cool for approximately 15 minutes.

Meanwhile, combine coconut milk or Rice Dream, cardamom, and rose water in a saucepan and simmer over low heat for 2 to 3 minutes, until fragrant. Let cool.

To serve, divide ricotta balls into 4 bowls (3 balls in each) and divide cooled coconut milk or Rice Dream evenly among the bowls, pouring it over the balls. Top with almond slivers and serve at room temperature.

Makes 4 servings

GINGER SNICKERDOODLES

These lightly sweetened cookies are rich in protein and great for the whole family as a snack or a treat.

    2 cups blanched almond flour
    ⅓ cup agave nectar or honey
    ¼ cup (½ stick) unsalted butter, softened, plus more for greasing
    2 tsp ground ginger
    1 tsp vanilla extract
    1 tsp ground cinnamon
    ⅛ tsp baking soda

Combine all ingredients in a food processor and blend well. Transfer dough to a small bowl, cover, and refrigerate for 30 minutes.

Preheat oven to 325°F. Lightly butter a baking sheet.

Form chilled dough into 20 small balls and then flatten balls into disks. Arrange disks on prepared baking sheet. Bake for 10 minutes, until lightly browned. Let cool and serve immediately. Store leftovers in an airtight container for up to 4 days.

Makes 20 cookies

APPLE STREUSEL

This recipe can easily be converted to a protein-rich breakfast; double the portion to start your day right. Note: For those of you new to almond flour, blanched almond flour will produce a much lighter texture. You can make your own in a food processor with blanched almonds. If you decide to use a store-bought almond flour, I like Honeyville Farms.

2 tbsp unsalted butter, for greasing the jars

Streusel Topping

1½ cups blanched almond flour

2 tbsp brown sugar

¼ cup (½ stick) unsalted butter, softened

1 tsp ground cinnamon

Apple Filling

3 apples, cored and chopped into ½-inch pieces

2 tbsp brown sugar

1 tsp ground cinnamon

½ tsp cardamom

¼ tsp ground cloves

Special equipment: 8 (4-oz) mason jars

Preheat oven to 350°F. Lightly butter the 8 mason jars.

For streusel, in a medium bowl, mix all ingredients by hand or with a hand mixer. Set aside.

For filling, in a medium bowl, combine all ingredients and mix well.

Divide apple mixture evenly among the 8 buttered mason jars. Top with ½ inch streusel topping, packing down firmly. Place mason jars on a baking sheet to prevent toppling over.

Bake for 25 to 30 minutes, until streusel topping is lightly browned. Serve warm.

Makes 8 servings

CRÈME BRÛLÉE

5 large egg yolks

½ cup granulated sugar, plus more for dusting

1 cup canned full-fat unsweetened coconut milk

1 vanilla bean, sliced lengthwise, seeds scraped out

Preheat oven to 300°F. Bring a large pot of water to a boil.

Combine all ingredients in a large bowl and blend with a hand mixer for 3 to 4 minutes, until thoroughly blended. Divide mixture among 4 crème brûlée ramekins.

Place ramekins in a ceramic baking dish and pour hot water into dish (around ramekins) until it comes halfway up the ramekins, making a water bath. Carefully transfer baking dish to oven and bake custards for about 40 minutes, until centers are still slightly loose.

Chill custards in refrigerator for at least 1 hour or up to 24 hours. Top custards with sugar and caramelize sugar with a kitchen torch. If you don't have a kitchen torch, place ramekins under a broiler set on high for 3 to 4 minutes, until sugar starts to brown.

Makes 4 servings

Acknowledgments

I am so thankful to have the support of my team at Grand Central—Jamie Raab, Sarah Pelz, and Matthew Ballast. Thank you, Stacey Glick, for being such an amazing agent, and for your constant cheers.

I have an incredible debt of gratitude to my staff at The Plan. I can't thank you enough for the daily laughs, the constant brainstorming, and always thinking outside the box. To my team—Marjorie Spitz, Cindy Hwang, Dr. Katie Reinholtz, Althea White, and Jill Jaclin—you have generous spirits and incredible dedication. Thank you for helping people all over the world heal.

Noah Fecks, thank you for incredible photographs that are as delightful as your spirit.

I want to thank the chefs who chose to celebrate food with brilliant simplicity—women like Alice Waters and Mollie Katzen, and two bright stars we lost recently, Marcella Hazan and Judy Rodgers. Thank you for keeping food clean, vibrantly healthy, and true to its roots.

This cookbook is written for healthy eaters everywhere. I hope it will help you make your kitchen and table more joyful. Of course this book is especially for my Planners, because I love you like nobody's business! Every day you inspire me with your stories, your belief in yourself, and your ability to heal. As always, I am sending you a big, big hug!

Appendix

Converting to Metrics

VOLUME MEASUREMENT CONVERSIONS

U.S.	Metric
¼ teaspoon	1.25 ml
½ teaspoon	2.5 ml
¾ teaspoon	3.75 ml
1 teaspoon	5 ml
1 tablespoon	15 ml
¼ cup	62.5 ml
½ cup	125 ml
¾ cup	187.5 ml
1 cup	250 ml

WEIGHT MEASUREMENT CONVERSIONS

U.S.	Metric
1 ounce	28.4 g
8 ounces	227.5 g
16 ounces (1 pound)	455 g

COOKING TEMPERATURE CONVERSIONS

Celsius/Centigrade	0°C and 100°C are arbitrarily placed at the melting and boiling points of water and standard to the metric system
Fahrenheit	Daniel Fahrenheit established 0°F as the stabilized temperature when equal amounts of ice, water, and salt are mixed.

To convert Fahrenheit to Celsius, subtract 32 and multiply by .5555—this formula:

$$C = (F - 32) \times 0.5555$$

So, for example, if you are baking at 350°F and want to know that temperature in Celsius, use this calculation:

$$C = (350 - 32) \times 0.5555 = 176.65°C$$

Bibliography

Teodoro Bottiglieri, "S-Adenosyl-L-methionine (SAMe): From the Bench to the Bedside—Molecular Basis of a Pleiotrophic Molecule," *American Journal of Clinical Nutrition* 76, no. 5 (2002): 1151S–57S.

Wen Boynton and Martin Floch, "New Strategies for the Management of Diverticular Disease: Insights for the Clinician," *Therapeutic Advances in Gastroenterology* 6, no. 3 (2013): 205–13, doi: 10.1177/1756283X13478679.

G. M. Bressa, "S-Adenosyl-L-Methionine (SAMe) as Antidepressant: Meta-Analysis of Clinical Studies," *Acta Neurologica Scandinavica Supplement* 154 (1994): 7–14.

Hae Young Chung, Matteo Cesari, Stephen Anton, Emanuele Marzetti, Silvia Giovannini, Arnold Young Seo, Christy Carter, Byung Pal Yu, and Christiaan Leeuwenburgh, "Molecular Inflammation: Underpinnings of Aging and Age-Related Diseases," *Ageing Research Reviews* 8, no. 1 (2009): 18–30, doi: 10.1016/j.arr.2008.07.002.

"Diverticular Disease of the Colon," *Harvard Men's Health Watch* 14, no. 8 (2010): 1–4.

Abbas Ali Jafari, Elham Khanpayah, and Hakimah Ahadian, "Comparison the Oral Candida Carriage in Type 2 Diabetic and Non Diabetics," *Jundishapur Journal of Microbiology* 6, no. 7 (2013): e8495, doi: 10.5812/jjm.8495.

Y. Lavrovsky, B. Chatterjee, R. A. Clark, and A. K. Roy, "Role of Redox-Regulated Transcription Factors in Inflammation, Aging and Age-Related Diseases," *Experimental Gerontology* 35 (2000): 521–32, doi: 10.1016/S0531-5565(00)00118-2.

Hirofumi Maruyama and Tetsuro Ikekawa, "Combination Therapy of Transplanted Meth-A Fibrosarcoma in BALB/c Mice with Protein-Bound Polysaccharide EA6 Isolated from Enokitake Mushroom *Flammulina velutipes* (W.Curt.:Fr.) Singer and Surgical

Excision," *International Journal of Medicinal Mushrooms* 7 (2005): 213–20, doi: 10.1615/IntJMedMushr.v7.i12.200.

National Institute of Diabetes and Digestive and Kidney Diseases, "Diverticular Disease," NIH Publication no. 13-1163 (September 2013): 1–10.

J. Craig Nelson, "S-Adenosyl Methionine (SAMe) Augmentation in Major Depressive Disorder," *American Journal of Psychiatry* 167, no. 8 (2010): 889–91, doi: 10.1176/appi.ajp.2010.10040627.

Paul Stamets, *Growing Gourmet and Medicinal Mushrooms*, 3rd ed. (Berkeley, CA: Ten Speed Press, 2000).

Stamets, "Notes on Nutritional Properties of Culinary-Medicinal Mushrooms," *International Journal of Medicinal Mushrooms* 7 (2005): 103–10, doi: 10.1615/IntJMedMushr.v7.i12.100.

H. Yin, Y. Wang, Y. Wang, T. Chen, H. Tang, and M. Wang, "Purification, Characterization and Immuno-Modulating Properties of Polysaccharides Isolated from *Flammulina velutipes* Mycelium," *The American Journal of Chinese Medicine* 38, no. 1 (2010): 191–204, doi: 10.1142/S0192415X10007750.

Index

About the Author

LYN-GENET RECITAS is the *New York Times* bestselling author of *The Plan*, a ground-breaking anti-inflammatory nutritional protocol. Her work has been featured on *The Dr. Oz Show*, *Fox News*, and in the *Huffington Post*. She has been a holistic nutritionist for over thirty years, studying nutritional therapy, holistic medicine, herbology, home-opathy, yoga, and shiatsu. Lyn-Genet and her team at The Lyn-Genet Plan have helped hundreds of thousands of men and women find easy, effective ways to lose weight, improve health, and reverse the aging process.